—C. Norman Shealy, MD, PhD, Author of *Pony Wisdom for the Soul* and Executive Producer of *Medical Renaissance—The Secret Code*

"Anyone interested in finding an effective, user-friendly, shortcut method for alleviating pain, anxiety and other forms of emotional distress, should learn Dr. Benor's method, WHEE. This is an abbreviated, ingenious combination of EMDR and EFT, and it is all spelled out in this wonderful book."

—Belleruth Naparstek, LISW, Author of *Invisible Heroes: Survivors of Trauma and How They Heal,* and Creator of the *Health Journeys Guided Imagery AudioSeries*

"Daniel Benor gently holds the reader's hand as he shows the way to fearlessly walk up to our pain, greet it, have gentle conversation, learn from it and then truly lessen or resolve the pain. WHEE is a gift one keeps enjoying forever, like a favorite drink in an ever-full bottle. Cheers!"

—Tapas Fleming, Founder, Tapas Acupressure Technique™ (TAT), www.tatlife.com

"Dr. Benor, a pioneer in wholistic healing, has achieved what great minds strive for—a system so elegantly simple that anyone can use it. Originated to help children and adults with pain and stress, 7 Minutes to Natural Pain Release *will show you not only how to relieve physical pain but also psychological pain and spiritual angst. Read. Apply. Enjoy. It is that easy!"*

—David Feinstein, Ph.D., Coauthor of *Personal Mythology* and *Promise of Energy Psychology*

"Dr. Benor articulates with superb clarity an original, scholarly guiding light into the world of pain. This book is for both neophytes and experienced clinicians on how to dialogue and extract the meaning of pain, providing powerful techniques for managing pain and creating health. I highly recommend this jewel of wisdom."

—Lee Pulos, PhD, ABPP, Author of *The Biology of Empowerment* and *The Power of Visualization*

Seven Minutes to Natural Pain Release

Pain is a Choice and Suffering Is Optional— WHEE for Tapping Your Pain Away

by Daniel J. Benor, MD

Wholistic Healing Publications
PO Box 76
Bellmawr, NJ 08099
www.wholhealpubs.com

Cataloging-in-Publication Data

Benor, Daniel J., MD
   7 minutes to natural pain release : pain is a choice and suffering is optional — WHEE
for tapping your pain away / by Daniel J. Benor, MD — 2nd ed.
      p. cm.
   Includes bibliographical references and index.
   ISBN 978-0-9819729-0-9
   1. Energy psychology. 2. Pain — Alternative treatment. 3. Mental healing. 4. Self-
help techniques. 5. Psychic trauma — Alternative treatment. I. Title. II. Title: Seven
minutes to natural pain release.
   RC489.E53B466 2009
   616.89 — dc22

First edition: Seven minutes to natural pain release: WHEE for tapping your pain
away — the revolutionary new self-healing method, by Daniel J. Benor, MD, Santa
Rosa, CA: Energy Psychology Press 2008.

Disclaimer: The techniques described in this book are intended as information for
therapists, not for self-treatment. If you are having stress problems, you should seek
the help of a therapist who can guide you in identifying and using
the techniques that will best suit your problems.

Cover design by Victoria Valentine
Photos on pages iv, 136 and 225 by Debbie Lerman
Typesetting by Karin Kinsey
Typeset in Cochin and Adobe Garamond
Printed in USA
2nd Edition

10 9 8 7 6 5 4 3 2

WHEE

Whole Health—Easily and Effectively®

AKA

Wholistic Hybrid derived from EMDR
and EFT

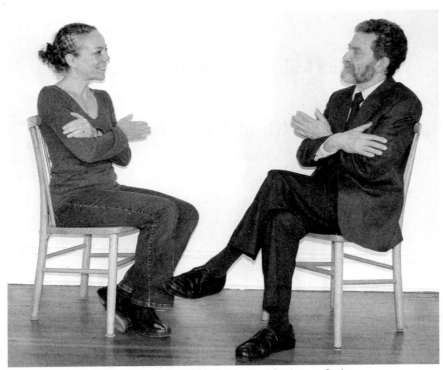
Dr. Benor teaching WHEE using the butterfly hug.

Contents

Acknowledgments

I am grateful to Francine Shapiro, who developed EMDR, and to Gary Craig, who developed EFT. Both methods have been enormously helpful to me personally and have helped countless clients, who benefited when I practiced these therapies as they were taught and afterward, when I combined elements derived from EMDR and EFT into WHEE.

I owe a great debt of thanks to Asha Nahoma Clinton, PhD, who in one little gesture, in November of 2000, birthed WHEE in my awareness. I had mentioned to her that my compliance rate was low with children and their parents using EFT. Asha tapped her eyebrows alternately across the bridge of her nose, saying, "You can get the same results just using these points." As she did that, I said to myself, "But that's EMDR!"

I am grateful to all the wonderful people who have been open in telling me about their experiences of pains of many varieties. These brave souls have dug into the caves where all sorts of personal issues were buried and have released them with WHEE, thereby benefiting not only themselves but also me and many others who have suffered from physical and psychological pains and learned from their examples.

I am deeply grateful to many wise counselors, healers, and clients who have helped me on my personal path of healing. I am particularly indebted to Wendy Hurwitz, MD, Martina Steiger, ThD, Ruth Sewell, PhD, RN, Mary Ann Wallace, MD, and Laurel Thom, each of whom has been incredibly helpful to me on various occasions in my process of peeling the onion of life. I am no different from readers of this book. At times it is as challenging for me as for anyone else to deal with difficult issues—to uncover and unravel the tangle of events, my responses to them, and my defenses against dealing with pains that I have experienced.

I am grateful to countless authors and conference presenters who have enriched my appreciation for the diversity of the human condition and the endless variations on the themes of healing they have explored and developed. High on my list, but certainly not exclusive, are Lawrence LeShan (*The Medium, The Mystic, and The Physicist* and *Alternate Realities*), Eckart Tolle (*The Power of Now* and *A New Earth*); Larry Dossey (*Space, Time, and Medicine*), and Bernie Siegel (*Love, Medicine, and Miracles*).

I am grateful for the turns of events that led to this second edition of *Seven Minutes to Natural Pain Release*, which is a very slight revision of its first edition predecessor. The most notable change is the brief discussion of using WHEE to address the collective post-traumatic stress disorder of humanity. The other changes are notes on the choices involved in our pain experiences, as reflected in the new subtitle for this edition, "Pain Is A Choice and Suffering Is Optional."

I am grateful to the Infinite Source for choreographing my life on a path of healing—both personal and professional. The wounds I experienced growing up in my birth family were sufficiently deep to require healing, yet not so severe as to be incapacitating. I would also not have found my way to WHEE without the pain of disillusionment in my chosen profession of psychiatry. WHEE has helped me with the stress of leaving a practice that has shifted over the years from being all psychotherapy to being almost all medications.

I am grateful for the positive space in which I find myself, with the help of WHEE—developing ever-deeper levels of patience, trust, and spiritual awareness.

Introduction

If you think you cannot do something that you can, the belief itself prevents you from accomplishing the task, either because you never try it in the first place or because you have blocked yourself by your beliefs.

—Deena Zalkind Spear

Welcome to the WHEE method for potent, quick, and easy pain relief. In opening this page in your life, you are entering a doorway to deep transformation on all levels of your being.

This book will be an enormous help to you if you feel that you are up against a wall of pain, frustrations with medications and other treatments, and the anxieties, annoyance, anger, and depression that often accompany pain. It will also help you with any other issues in your life that you would like to feel better about. You are joining the many people who have used WHEE with astounding, rapid relief of physical and psychological pains—even those that have been present for a long time.

WHEE gives you the skills to transmute pain and suffering on any and all levels of your being. The more you explore the uses of WHEE, the more you will grow to be the person you want to be, and to leave behind whatever you wish to release.

If you are a therapist who uses other Energy Psychology techniques or EMDR, you will also find this book helpful because you can easily shift to using WHEE or might choose to adapt many of the approaches I have learned from using WHEE to your own methods.

If you are a caregiver new to these innovative methods of helping people to heal themselves, you will find it pleasantly easy to learn this potent, rapidly effective method for self-healing. You will likewise find it satisfying to be able to help people in your practice to learn and use WHEE.

WHEE is elegantly simple. People who are successful in shifting issues that have plagued them for years will often say, "I still can't believe I'm free of that problem. I don't understand how a method that is so simple could achieve complete pain relief when nothing else was able to help me over the long, long time I've suffered with this issue!"

> At a conference in Zurich on healing, a woman volunteered to demonstrate to the audience how WHEE worked for pains in both shoulders that had limited her severely in raising her arms for two years. Within minutes, she was free of these pains and a bit incredulous about this. Asked what she would like to do, now that she could move her arms, she said, "I'd like to give you a big hug! And then a hug for my husband, who is sitting over there."

WHEE is so effective because it helps beyond the direct release of pains. WHEE quickly identifies any blocks or resistances to releasing pains. These blocks are *meta-rules* we develop out of anxieties and fears about releasing hurts that lie buried in our unconscious mind. These beliefs persist, telling us that we still cannot handle or tolerate the feelings we buried at the time we experienced them. WHEE helps to dismantle these beliefs so that they no longer block the release of the buried hurts. Much more on this in Chapter 3.

We all know the experience of pain. It hurts! We don't like it and will do just about anything to avoid having it.

> *Illness is the doctor to whom we pay most heed;*
> *to kindness, to knowledge we make promises only;*
> *to pain we obey.*
>
> —Marcel Proust

You might be surprised to know that pain is actually an extremely complicated subject. Numerous factors can initiate, perpetuate, worsen, or lessen your perceptions of and responses to your pain. These range from your genetic and cultural inheritance through many types of physical and psychological factors. These are discussed in Chapter 1. Spiritual ways of filtering and dealing with the experience of pain are discussed in Chapter 6.

Your body and mind are intimately linked with each other. You may find the same pain to be a very different experience, depending upon your perceptions of it in various contexts. You may have noticed that if you stub your toe on the foot of your bed in the morning it may not hurt as much as if you stub your toe on the exact same place at night. When you are fresh and energetic, looking toward a new day of activities, the pain in your stubbed toe sits within different frames of reference than when you are tired and ready for sleep.

Not only is the physical perception of pain a variable factor, but your psychological relationships with your pain can change its intensity and your interactions with it. Chapter 2 explores varieties of psychological factors that may influence your pain.

Pain is often a message from our inner self, spoken through the symptoms of our body. Physical and emotional pains, along with other experiences of adversity, are sometimes signals chosen by our inner wisdom to pause and reconsider what we are doing or not doing with our lives. Many have told me that as much as they would not have chosen to have their pains, the experiences of dealing with the pains have actually helped them in many ways. They have reassessed their priorities, goals, work commitments, relationships, and leisure pleasures, treating themselves more gently and generously than ever before. Many have also found themselves calling upon and connecting with a higher power in their lives, finding that this not only helps with the pains, but is deeply satisfying and enriching—beyond anything they had ever anticipated or experienced before. Chapter 6 shares some possibilities of ways that you can invite more of this deeply satisfying personal spirituality into your life.

"Sally" came to me recently for help with her right thumb, which she had injured in a snowmobile accident a month earlier.

There was no fracture and the pain continued to be excruciating when she was writing.

Dialoguing with her pain, she came to realize it was telling her to listen more to her intuition. The accident had occurred after she followed her husband across a lake, despite her inner feeling that this was unsafe.

Sally had already started listening to this message, though this was not a conscious awareness. Shortly after the snowmobile accident, her husband was driving with her as passenger. He wanted to pass a truck, and Sally (uncharacteristically for her) strongly urged him to hold back. He heeded her suggestion and they avoided what would have certainly been a serious head-on collision.

Sally's pain was significantly reduced from this dialogue. (More on this in Chapter 4.)

People often ask me, "But how can something so simple work so deeply and quickly and thoroughly, even clearing pains that have been present for many years?" Theories to explain WHEE are considered in Chapter 7.

I developed WHEE as a system for dealing with pains and stresses of all kinds, including tension headaches, migraines, backaches, pains after injuries and surgery, arthritis, stomachaches, irritable bowel syndromes, chronic fatigue syndrome, fibromyalgia, cancer, and more. Chapter 4 details how you can use WHEE for rapid, deep, and often permanent relief of pain. If you have chronic pains, however, I caution you to read Chapter 1 before jumping in to use WHEE.

Pain may be a signal from the body that we are "uptight" over a stressful situation and are in distress. We may be unaware of what it is that is stressing us, and this is the way our unconscious mind chooses to grab our attention to seek out and deal with our distress. Chronic pain may take on a life of its own, leading us to behave in ways that actually perpetuate or even increase the pain and make it difficult to release. It is important to consider such possibilities carefully before working on removing the pain. Chapter 5 considers these and many other issues around the treatment of pains—acute and chronic.

Grateful people who use WHEE report that in addition to helping with pain, it also has helped them with emotional pains; anxieties; fears; phobias; post-traumatic stress disorders (PTSDs); angers; insomnia; reducing side effects and the need for medications; dealing with cravings—for sweets, food, drugs, thrills; motion sickness and morning sickness of pregnancy; allergies; and weight loss. Relationships, social issues, performance anxieties, low self-confidence, and low self-esteem have all responded to WHEE, as well as family members' anxieties and distress.

I, myself, am as grateful as anyone else for the benefits of WHEE. This method has helped me deal with various stresses, including the stress of working in medical systems that severely limited my scope for helping people. It has helped me with my own headaches, post-injury and post-surgery pains, and pains that arose from my unconscious mind as messages to explore deeper, unconscious issues.

WHEE was born from my frustrations as a psychiatrist. I have always been passionate about doing psychotherapy. I studied psychology as an undergraduate, then endured the challenges of medical school, with a year's break for a National Institutes of Mental Health (NIMH) research fellowship in psychiatry and for regrouping my battered energies. I trained as a psychiatrist from 1967–1973, when psychiatry was mostly psychotherapy (with two intervening years in the Air Force during the Vietnam War). Since then, managed care has squeezed psychiatrists towards medication management and away from psychotherapy.

While I resisted prescribing medications exclusively, it is pretty difficult to do much psychotherapy in a 15–30 minute medication visit once a month—the amount of time allowed in the U.S. under managed care. I constantly sought to develop ways of providing psychotherapy along with the medications, but was unable within my limited timeframe to use the psychodynamic approaches I was taught as a psychiatric resident. These were fine when I had had 50 minutes once or twice a week, but impossible to use in the much more limited timeframes I was allowed under managed care.

Eye Movement Desensitization and Reprocessing (EMDR) was a blessing to me as well as to my clients.[1] This very simple technique

[1] See www.emdr.com.

involves alternating right and left stimulation of the body, back and forth, while focusing on feelings (often attached to an experience or issue) that one would like to change. Doing EMDR repeatedly can reduce and eliminate negative feelings fairly quickly if they are associated with a single traumatic experience. EMDR will also help with traumas such as chronic abuse, but this may take weeks, months, or years, depending on the severity of the traumatic experiences. Once the negative feelings are released, a positive statement is installed, using a similar process, to replace the negatives that have been released.

I was able to use EMDR with clients who had anxieties, phobias, and even with PTSDs. I also used EMDR to de-stress myself.

It is recommended that EMDR should be done only in the therapist's presence. This is to prevent being overwhelmed by intense emotional releases that can occur during treatment. This was a severe limit on the benefits I could offer my clients with EMDR.

I then learned to use the Emotional Freedom Technique (EFT) developed by Gary Craig[2] and other Meridian Based Therapies (MBTs). In EFT and related therapies one taps or presses a finger at a series of acupressure points on the face, chest, and hand, while reciting an affirmation. Similar to EMDR in its effects, the negative feelings are released as one repeats this process. Classical EFT does not install positives to replace the negatives that have been released. Because it does not evoke intense emotional releases, EFT can be used as self-healing outside the therapist's office.

EFT was very helpful to those who used it. However, many complained that they could not remember the long series of acupressure points they needed to use in EFT. This was all the more problematic if they were upset, because when they were anxious and flustered they had even more difficulties recalling the procedure.

The Basics of WHEE

In an introductory workshop by Asha Nahoma Clinton on Matrix Therapy, she observed that alternating tapping the eyebrows on either side of the bridge of the nose while reciting the affirmation works just as

---

[2] See www.emofree.com.

well as the entire series of EFT points. I realized immediately that this
is the same as the right-left body stimulation of EMDR. Ever conscious
of my time limitations, I immediately started exploring this hybrid
approach, which combines aspects of EMDR and EFT. I now call this
the Wholistic Hybrid derived from EMDR and EFT, or WHEE. A
more user-friendly name is Whole Health — Easily and Effectively.

EMDR suggests the use of a "butterfly hug" as one of its self-treatment interventions, particularly for children. To do this, one's arms are
crossed so that the hands rest on the biceps muscles, tapping alternately
on each arm. I often have children and parents use the butterfly hug
with the affirmation instead of tapping at the eyebrows. Many find the
self-hug comforting, in addition to being highly effective in combination
with the affirmation.

Affirmations are another important feature of WHEE. Here is a
generic one, adapted from EFT:

> "Even though I have this [pain/anxiety/stress/other symp-
> tom], I wholly and completely love and accept myself [or use
> whatever strong positive statement suits you best at the time
> you need it]."

Prior to and following each use of WHEE, it is helpful to assess the
strength of the negative feeling you want to address. The most commonly used assessment is the *Subjective Units of Distress Scale* (SUDS), in
which the feeling is located along a scale from zero (not bothering you
at all) to 10 (the worst it could possibly feel).

After tapping for a few minutes, check the SUDS again. It will usually go down. Repeat the assessing and tapping until it is zero.

Once the SUDS level is down to zero, it is helpful to install a *replacement positive statement* to take the place of the negative issue that has been
released. For instance, if you have released an anxiety over your next
doctor's visit, you might start tapping and say something like: "I can
have my examination, any tests, and treatment and feel comfortable and
good about it, and I love and accept myself, wholly and completely."
Prior to starting to install the replacement positive, and after each round
of WHEE to strengthen it, you will find it helpful to check how strongly
you believe the replacement positive statement to be true, where zero

is "not at all" and 10 is "it couldn't be stronger or firmer." This is the Subjective Units of Success Scale (SUSS).

I find the combination of EMDR and EFT more potent and effective than either alone. Chapter 3 will introduce you to WHEE in much more detail, and will explain further about its many user-friendly benefits.

- WHEE has been hugely successful and enthusiastically accepted for several reasons:

- WHEE is elegantly simple and easy to learn.

- WHEE takes a fraction of the time that EFT and other MBTs require.

- WHEE can be taught in groups of any size in person, and in groups of up to ten on a telephone conference call. In the group setting participants can maintain privacy around sensitive issues they are working on, disclosing only the intensity of the feelings around issues they are addressing.

- WHEE allows for great flexibility in working on target problems within the session because it is so rapid. If a person has difficulties in lightening their pains and other problems, there is plenty of time in a session to explore alternative target symptoms or alternative methods of addressing these.

- WHEE is better accepted and the compliance outside the therapy room is much higher because of its rapid action and simplicity.

- WHEE is marvelously successful and rapidly effective for pains of all sorts, including tension headaches, migraines, stomach-aches, irritable bowel syndromes, backaches, pains after injuries and surgery, arthritis, cancer, chronic fatigue syndrome, fibromyalgia, and more.

- WHEE is excellent for allergies, though it may take several days to be effective for these.

- WHEE is tremendously empowering, as it is so simple and so rapidly effective in self-healing. People are very pleased to be able to help themselves, not having to rely as much on medications or interventions of a therapist, although the guidance of a therapist may facilitate the self-healing uses of WHEE.

- WHEE is a wholistic healing method that helps on every level of our being: body, emotions, mind, relationships (with other people and with the environment), and spirit.

Many more details for using WHEE will be discussed in Chapter 3, and further explanations for the success of WHEE are detailed in Chapter 7.

I suggest that you explore for yourself how the various elements of WHEE work for you. WHEE is so simple that you can follow the descriptions in this book and discover and enjoy its benefits immediately. You can know in your innermost being whether what I suggest is true and helpful for you, as it has been for countless others who have explored and benefited from WHEE.

My personal experience in six years of using WHEE has been that there is virtually no issue of feelings or thoughts that will fail to respond to the WHEE protocols. This is not a magic wand. It is, rather, like a vacuum cleaner that allows you to clear out old, dusty emotional and cognitive junk from the inner filing cabinets and closets where you stored them at times when you didn't want to deal with them or felt they were more than you could handle. At times, this old junk may resist your removing it. With practice, you will learn to understand your resistances and will then be able to address them through some variation of WHEE practices. This is not to claim that WHEE is a cure-all, but that it can at least ease nearly every issue and can completely alleviate the discomforts of many.

Numerous case examples are presented to illustrate various aspects of the WHEE process. Names and details have been altered to protect the anonymity of those described.

To illustrate how WHEE has helped me personally, I will share a series of clearings of my own residues of issues from my relationship with my mother. This illustrates a variety of WHEE applications for the same problem, and clarifies how a deep issue can be peeled, one layer of the onion at a time, as aspects of that issue rise to the surface of awareness.

No one shoe fits all, and no single approach is suitable or effective for addressing every type and variety of pain. However, in five years of offering a money-back guarantee in workshops in many countries around the world, I have only had one person claim a refund on the basis of having experienced no benefits whatsoever.

WHEE is adaptable to your specific needs and preferences. It is a scaffold that you can construct from the elements in this book to support and enhance your personal way of being. Choose those suggestions that feel right and which you find are helpful in reducing or eliminating your pain. Be aware, however, that an element that doesn't suit you today may be just right next week or next year.

WHEE will help you convert worries that feel unmanageable and burdensome into concerns that you can address appropriately.

One further clarification about WHEE here: WHEE is not going to help you *forget* anything negative that you have experienced. WHEE helps to release negative feelings and beliefs *about* what you have experienced. While the memories may remain, they will no longer have a negative charge to them when you replay old tapes of experiences and bring them up on the screen of your awareness. Many people do find that the intensity of the memory fades as the negative emotions and beliefs connected with the memories are reduced or eliminated. When this happens, some report that it is then difficult to bring the memories up on the screen of their mind. They commonly report, "It's like the colors and sounds have faded and it's hard to see or hear them any more."

You may find yourself drawn to skip around in this book to whichever chapters interest you most. This is fully in line with the spirit of WHEE, which encourages each person to adapt the WHEE methods to their own individual situations and needs.

Many of the observations about WHEE presented in this book are equally applicable to other Energy Psychology therapies. The fact that WHEE is such a rapidly effective intervention has made it easier to sort out the various elements that produce changes in this form of self-healing treatment.

There are further helpful references at the end of this book, as well as a glossary to help you with unfamiliar terms. If you are interested in further reading, you may wish to explore the WHEE workbook, available at www.wholistichealingresearch.com. I also offer experiential phone and in-person workshops to teach WHEE.

1

Understanding
Pain

Your pain is the breaking of the shell that encloses your understanding.

—Khalil Gibran

We all know what pain feels like. We may have cut ourselves with a kitchen knife or the edge of a piece of paper; stubbed a toe or barked a shin on a piece of furniture; or may even have fallen and bruised our flesh or broken our bones. Various illnesses may have been accompanied by pains, sometimes for many months and years at a time.

Pain is no fun. We do everything we can to avoid it. When we feel pain, we often feel anxieties as well—particularly with more severe or long-lasting pains. If pains continue, we may feel emotionally debilitated and may even sink into depression. At other times we may become frustrated and angry. With any of these negative reactions, we may become 'up tight' and thereby worsen our pain

Pain is our body's way of telling us something is wrong and needing our attention. This is a help in survival. If we've injured a leg or an arm or some other part of our body, our tissues need time to repair themselves. Pain lets us know about the injury and reminds us to be gentle with the injured parts so they can recover more readily.

Conventional Explanations for Pain

There is a theory which states that if ever anyone discovers exactly what the Universe is for and why it is here, it will instantly disappear and be replaced by something even more bizarre and inexplicable. There is another which states that this has already happened.

—Douglas Adams

Conventional Western medical considerations of pain seek to analyze various components of our pain experience. This is called *reductionism*—studying smaller and smaller pieces of a problem on the assumption that if each component is fully understood then it will be easier to address the whole problem and, hopefully, to cure it.

Within this model there are many ways that something might go wrong and cause pain:

1. Pain perception is initiated by stimulation of nerve endings in the various organs of the body. Sources of stimulation can include:

   - *Mechanical factors*—Trauma ranging from chronic external pressure to acute blows or cuts; internal trauma from heavy or chronic, repetitive use of the musculoskeletal system beyond its natural capacities (as in repetitive strain injury); and swelling or other deformity of organs and tissues from factors such as excessive body fluid (edema), infection, and direct trauma to nerves.

   - *Chemical or metabolic factors*—Caustic external substances or toxins that damage tissues or cause muscle spasms; and accumulations of physiological toxins within the body.

   - *Thermal or electromagnetic stimulation*—Reactions range from unpleasant sensations, through muscle spasms, to destruction of tissues.

   - *Infections*—Direct inflammation of nerves or indirect pain via swelling of tissues and organs.

   - *Neoplasms*—Tumors with invasions of tissues and nerves, or indirect pain via swelling of, or encroachment upon, tissues and organs, especially nerves that are sensitive and bones that have no flexibility or "give."

- *Degenerative factors* —wearing out of tissues and joint surfaces, with pain felt as the body "complains" about overuse or deterioration of the cartilage.

- *Immune system responses* —Swelling or inflammation of tissues because of allergic reactions that produce inflammation (rheumatoid arthritis is included here because it is thought to be caused by autoimmune reactions).

- *Neurophysiological factors* —Malfunctions of the brain and peripheral nervous systems, either producing sensations of pain due to malfunctions in pain nerves or leading to tension in muscles, which eventually tire or spasm, producing pain, which in turn creates a vicious circle of psychological irritability, more tension, and more pain (discussed later in this chapter).

- *Psychological factors* —Muscle spasms from tension or conditioned responses; metaphors for emotional problems that are expressed through muscle tensions; and *phantom limb* phenomena following amputations (all of these are discussed in greater detail in Chapter 2).

2. Pain perception is variable between different people. Pain is more than a simple chain of cause and effect of physical and psychological relationships. One person may have little reaction to a given painful stimulus, while another may writhe in agony under the (apparently) same stimulus or condition. Psychological factors influencing pain perception may involve:

- *Innate differences in pain thresholds* —One person may have lesser or greater sensitivity to certain stimuli than another.

- *General state of the nervous system (whether affected by tiredness, anxiety, or other emotional factors)* —This may relate to altered sensitivity thresholds, or to the amount of energy a person has for coping with the added stress of pain.

- *Specific psychological factors* —For example, people may tolerate post-surgical pain well if they know that the operation has resulted in a cure of their illness, or they may tolerate the same pain poorly if they hear that the surgery brought only a diagnosis of incurable disease.

- *Family and/or cultural conditionings* — These teach a person to be stoic or vociferous in responding to pain.

- *Attention factors* — At the height of an emergency or exciting situation, a person might not feel pain despite a severe injury. Only later, when attention is focused on the wound, is the pain perceived. Hypnosis may similarly decrease pain.

- *Mood factors* — These may influence responsivity to pain (anxiety and depression may increase pain, tranquility and joy decrease it).

- *Rewards associated with the expression of pain* — These may influence the frequency of its occurrence and the severity of its expression.

- *Phantom limb phenomena* — Persistence of perceptions in a part of the body (limb, breast) that has been amputated, often associated with pains that are experienced as though the limb were still present.

- *Fantasy pains* — Sensations seemingly created by the mind, where no objective causes can be identified. These may be body metaphor equivalents for anxieties, emotions, traumatic experiences, and psychotic misperceptions and misinterpretations of reality. (More on these later in this chapter.)

3. Transpersonal or spiritual awareness may contribute to how we experience and comprehend our pains.

   - Pain may be experienced and interpreted as a stimulus for people to pray, or to question why we are suffering. We may look deep within ourselves for answers, or ask God for help in understanding and dealing with our injury or illness. At the very least, pain may be our unconscious mind's way of forcing us to take a break from stresses or lifestyles that are in some way harmful.

      Many people who have serious health issues come to feel that their illness led them to re-examine their lives, and to make enormously enriching decisions for better relationships and more emotionally satisfying and rewarding careers, not to mention healthier lifestyles. This life-transforming process may come as a response to the physical challenges that force them to face their mortality and ask questions about the meaning of life.

- We may come to feel a spiritual causality that underlies and guides major life challenges, sensing that we might have been deliberately invited or pushed into such experiences—by our higher self, by spirit or angelic guides, or by the Infinite Source—as a way of deepening our spiritual quest in life.

    Pain may be related to lessons chosen by our higher self or soul for our spiritual growth. When we are free of pain we tend to be complacent and coast along, enjoying life but not learning very much. When we are in pain we are challenged to find new solutions to our problems, to plumb the depths of our being, and to push beyond the limits of our ordinary capabilities and awareness.

- Pain may be a residual from a previous incarnation, in which case it invites us to explore this dimension of our existence and to resolve ancient emotional scars.

Wholistic Ways of Addressing Pain

The part can never be well unless the whole is well.

—Plato

Wholisitc healing accepts that the study of individual components of pain, as above, is helpful but then goes several steps further:

- The subject of assessment and treatment is the person who has the pains, not just the pains that the person has.

- Pain is viewed as the individual expression of people's state of being in the world, within themselves as well as in their relationships with others, with their environment, and with their spiritual connections.

- Multiple aspects of the components of pain mentioned above are relevant in the study of each person's experience of pain. Wholistic healing addresses many factors contributing to pain.

Each person's experience of pain is unique. While there are certainly commonalities between one tension headache and another, each individual will feel and interpret the experience of pain through the filter of her own personal combination of all of the factors listed above. Therefore, approaches to addressing each person's pain are best when they are specifically tailored for that individual.

This is not to say that common problems will not respond to similar treatments. Aspirin may be perfectly adequate to deal with a headache. This is the usual way that conventional medicine treats pains of all sorts, and much of the time it works. We can treat our own headaches similarly.

There are several problems with this approach, however. The first is that medicating a pain is symptomatic treatment. This is usually helpful if the pain is an occasional, temporary experience. However, if the pain occurs frequently or is present constantly, then treating it symptomatically is similar to screwing the lid on a pot to keep it from boiling over rather than turning down the fire under the pot.

The second problem with this approach is that all medications cause side effects. Pain medications can produce drowsiness, mental fuzziness, nausea, ulcers, constipation and, as with all drugs, allergic reactions.

The third is that pain medications can interact with other medications, sometimes causing severe problems. As an example, aspirin can interact with anticoagulants (blood thinners) given to people who have had problems with blood clots, increasing beyond the range of safety the time it takes for blood to clot.

The fourth serious concern is that pain medications can be fatal. Aside from fatal allergic reactions, accidental overdoses may occur. Aspirin is still the most common drug overdose killer in early childhood, even though bottles are limited to 36 tablets in the US in the hopes of preventing this unfortunate problem. In rare cases, if given after chickenpox or other viral illnesses, aspirin can cause the Reye syndrome, which is often fatal. Other pain medications, such as the NSAID family of drugs, can cause fatal ulcers, heart attacks, and strokes.

If you are still inclined to take pain medications, you might consider the following statistics: Over 100,000 people die annually in the US alone from medications that are properly prescribed and used. Combining these with medical errors and misused medications, about 250,000 people die annually in the US. *This makes medical care the third leading cause of death*—ahead of auto accidents, violent crimes, and most diseases (other than cancer and heart disease). Pain medicines have been among the more common contributors to these deaths.

While this book focuses on WHEE, I in no way mean to imply that this modality is the be-all and end-all of therapies for pains. I honor the methods and traditions of other holistic therapies, including the many variations of Energy Psychology, acupuncture and its derivatives, homeopathy, imagery, and further therapies detailed in my books, *Healing Research, Volumes 2, Professional and Popular Editions.*

Seeking the causes of pains is like participating in a mystery theater production. All the clues are usually there, but it is up to us to identify them and put together the causal pattern that is creating the pain. This is often more challenging than treating the pain itself.

Even when the pain is caused by clear physical problems, there is almost always a psychological component that makes the pain worse or less tolerable than it might be. The very nature of pain is to make us uptight, which immediately makes it harder to tolerate the pain. Behind the pain there are often contributing psychological factors, as well. All of these issues will be discussed in the following chapters.

Psychological problems associated with pain respond very readily to WHEE. Within minutes, it is possible to release old hurts, anxieties, fears, angers, and other issues that contribute to the pain.

Addressing the pain with WHEE can relieve physical problems as well as psychological ones.

> In a WHEE workshop in Mexico, a woman asked for help with her arthritis. Her hands were so affected that she had not been able to bend any of her fingers for many months. We did an experiment, having her focus the WHEE on her right index finger. Within minutes, she was able to bend that finger but not any of the others.
>
> * * *
>
> A secretary in my office suffered with migraines so severe that her doctor had scheduled her for brain scans to rule out a tumor or other physical problem. Using WHEE, she was able to stop her present migraine immediately, and to eliminate further attacks permanently within a few weeks.

How WHEE can influence the body in these ways is unclear. We know, however, from studies of hypnotherapy and other approaches that the mind has vast self-healing capacities that we often fail to appreciate.[1]

The advantages of WHEE are:

- WHEE is a self-healing method that you will always have available to you.

- WHEE is rapidly effective, reducing and eliminating pain within minutes in many cases.

- WHEE addresses the roots of problems.

- WHEE is safe.

- WHEE allows you to install positive responses to your outer and inner life experiences, to replace the negatives you have released.

If you're the kind of person who likes to read ahead in a mystery novel, you may wish to skip to Chapter 3 to learn further details of how WHEE works. Otherwise, you may wish to continue with Chapter 2 to learn more about psychological factors in pain.

---

[1] For detailed discussions of the mind-body and body-mind connection, see *Healing Research, Volume 2: How Can I Heal What Hurts?* or the professional edition of the same book, *Consciousness, Bioenergy and Healing.*

2

Psychological Factors
in Pain

*Pain is such an uncomfortable feeling that even a tiny amount of it
is enough to ruin every enjoyment.*

— Will Rogers

I
n order to give you a better understanding of the complex elements
of physical pain, let me first expand on its various components. I
will then discuss psychological pains that may be manifested into
physical issues. Finally, we will consider the complex ways in which
pains may be woven into our lives, making them a challenge to understand and to deal with.

Components of Physical Pain

Pain is only valuable once you know that you've learned from it.

— Mary Tyler Moore

Pain is more than a simple chain of cause and effect of physical
problems and psychological responses to these. In fact, *pain perception
is highly variable between different people.* One person may have lesser or
greater sensitivity to certain stimuli than another.

Our genes seem to contribute to these differences. This has been
confirmed in infants who demonstrate different thresholds for responses to all stimulation, including touch, sound, and visual cues. You may
know people, as I have, who react strongly to pain and other issues

and situations, and conversely, people who are more likely to suffer in silence.

Our family and culture also contribute to how demonstrative we are in expressing our pain. When I was in training in obstetrics in medical school, the nurses cautioned me not to over-treat women of Latin cultures with pain medications if they were crying out loudly with labor pains. In their culture, this is the norm during labor. In contrast, women of Anglo-American descent are much more muted in their expressions of pain during labor. Had I not had this warning, I might have given the Latin women heavy doses of medications that could have slowed their labor and interfered with delivery.

Personal Psychological Factors

Psychological factors unique to the individual often contribute to the intensity of pain responses. These relate to how we have learned to respond to stress and tensions in our lives. Many people tense their bodies when they are frightened or even if they are just worried. When muscles are tense over a period of time they may get locked in painful spasms of tightness.

This is a common cause of neck and back pains. People who work at a table that is too low for their height may bend their backs and necks for long hours. Their muscles may complain through spasms of pain, asking for relief. I have had numbers of students suffer this way from poor posture while leaning over for long hours to do their homework, either at a table or with a computer; as well as kitchen and factory workers who spend long hours bent over a work table, and teachers who spend long hours grading papers. The solution for many of these pains is to adjust the height of the work surface.

Without realizing this, however, such experiences of muscle spasms may later predispose us to pains in these same muscles when we are tensed up from tiredness, stress, and worries. Muscles that have once been stressed to the point of spasms become sensitized and may be the first part of our body to alert us if we become tense in later situations.

Words that we use to express our tensions and frustrations may also sensitize particular parts of our bodies to become tense when we are "uptight." If a person repeatedly and emphatically says, "What a pain in the neck this is!" then their neck may respond by getting tensed up to the point of spasming whenever that person becomes frustrated or angry. With increased frequency or intensity of psychological tensions, their neck may go into spasm.

Here are a few other common expressions that have similar effects:[1]

- "My head is bursting with facts I have to remember!"

- "I keep swallowing down my anger!"

- "My guts are in an uproar over this worry!"

- "The lecture I had from my boss sure tightened my sphincters!"

Metaphors such as these may sensitize these parts of the body to tensions. In later situations of stress, these parts may then be the first to go into spasm again.

When I repress my emotion my stomach keeps score.

—John Enoch Powell

Generalized Tension

The general state of tension in our nervous system can increase or decrease our susceptibility to pains. When we are hungry, tired, frustrated, angry, or in any other way out of sorts or upset, our general level of irritability makes us less tolerant of pain. Conversely, when we are centered, calm, and at peace with ourselves and the world, our pain is nested in this tranquility and we feel it less or are at least less bothered by it.

Specific Psychological Factors

Many contextual psychological factors may predispose us to feel more or less pain. For example, stress and anxiety in any forms may heighten our responses to pain:

- It is well known in conventional medicine that distracting a person from looking at the injection needle as it is going in will lessen pain.

- Being totally focused on another issue may lessen or even prevent our feeling any pain at all. At the height of an emergency or

---

[1] Excerpted from a long list in *Healing Research, Volume 2.*

exciting situation (accident, battlefront engagement, sports event), while engrossed in achieving some immediate objective, a person might not feel pain despite a severe injury. Only later, when attention is focused on the wound, is the pain perceived. People who have a goal to work toward may focus all their attention on this and even deliberately ignore their pain, subsequently finding that they also feel the pain less.

- Having surgery in an unfamiliar setting, with strangers ministering to our needs at a time when we are helpless and vulnerable creates anxieties that can worsen the surgical outcomes, including increasing pain. With children, in particular, it is now standard practice in many hospitals to conduct tours of the operating theater prior to surgery, to familiarize them with their surroundings and lessen anxieties and stress.

- Receiving a diagnosis for the cause of our pain, even when we don't fully understand what the diagnosis means, removes anxieties about the unknown and reduces pain.

- Anticipatory anxieties of knowing that recurrent pains are likely to be severe for a period of time may make us tense and therefore subject to feeling pains more acutely. This is particularly true of people with migraines or people with severe chronic pains whose medications are not completely controlling the pain between medication doses.

Previous unpleasant experiences that resonate with our current situation may predispose us to more pain. Having had a difficult childbirth, a particularly painful dental extraction, an accident or prolonged wait in an emergency room where it took a long time to get pain relief, and other such traumas may leave us with residues of negative feelings and anticipations that increase our sensitivity to pain in a later, similar situation. I also have seen some people who had secondary traumas from the experiences of others who were close to them, or from seeing particularly painful or gruesome scenes in the media that predisposed them to react more strongly to their own pain on a later occasion that resembled in some ways what they had seen. One particularly useful method for uncovering such primary or inciting resonances is to connect with the unconscious mind through muscle testing.[2]

---

[2] The process for muscle testing is explained in detail in Chapter 3.

Mood Factors and Tiredness

Our general physical and emotional states may influence responsivity to pain. Anxiety, fear, and depression may increase pain, while tranquility and joy may decrease it.

You may notice that these factors overlap broadly with one another. This is because we tend to subdivide human experiences into small territories for easier exploration, when they are actually all interconnected. Mood and tiredness factors may influence our psychological and body tensions as one mechanism for influencing our pain sensitivity. However, they may make their own contributions to our pain as well.

The Pain/Gain Dichotomy

Rewards associated with the expression of pain may influence the frequency of its occurrence and the intensity of its expression. A person who unconsciously enjoys some benefit (secondary gain) from a pain, such as avoidance of unpleasant tasks or extra attention from family members, is likely to experience more pain. People who anticipate compensation following accidents are likely to relinquish their pains slowly, if at all.

> *I enjoy convalescence. It is the part that makes illness worthwhile.*
>
> —George Bernard Shaw

Phantom Limb Pain

Pain, or other sensations, may manifest as a persistence of perceptions in a part of the body (limb, breast) that has been amputated, and is often associated with pains that are experienced as though the body part were still present. Paraplegics (paralyzed from the waist down) may have phantom limb pains even when their spinal cords have been completely cut so that no ordinary sensations are felt from beyond the level of the nerves that were cut. Similarly, phantom limb sensations may be reported by people who were born without limbs.

Pains of Unknown Origins

Particularly torturous to those who have the misfortune to experience them are pains of unknown origin. One of these is fibromyalgia, a chronic condition that can include aching pains all over the body, including headaches. Adding to the torture of these pains is the torture of family, friends and physicians who may be skeptical about the reality of the pain, as there are no objective findings to validate them.

Fibromyalgia is associated with many of the same symptoms as chronic fatigue syndrome, including severe, chronic, debilitating tiredness that may make it impossible to even get out of bed; depression; mental fuzziness (often called *brain fog*); insomnia; and multiple allergies to foods and environmental chemicals. Fibromyalgia pains are worsened with exertion that exceeds a person's tolerance, but lessened with regular exercise that is gentle and not stressful. WHEE can help with many of these symptoms, particularly the pain, insomnia, and allergies. Other therapies that can help also include acupuncture, applied kinesiology, meditation, wholistic allergy treatments, and nutritional consultations regarding allergies.

Fantasy Pains

Some painful sensations are seemingly created by the mind, where no objective causes can be identified. Because fibromyalgia pains, for instance, may come on gradually and last for years, and because there is no objective medical test that can confirm or rule out its presence, some doctors question whether this is not a fantasy pain. Regardless of how they are described by Western medicine, however, such pains should not be dismissed as isolated figments of a person's imagination. Rather, they may be body metaphor equivalents for anxieties, emotions, traumatic experiences, and psychotic misperceptions and misinterpretations of reality. Some of these can be helped with WHEE, while others require more in-depth, long-term therapies.

Adapting to Pain

It has been said that "time heals all wounds." I do not agree. The wounds remain. In time, the mind, protecting its sanity, covers them with scar tissue and the pain lessens. But it is never gone.

—Rose Kennedy

Let's face it: having pain is no fun. It may change our lives from what we consider "normalcy" to being in an illness mode, from being carefree to having to be cautious and careful so that we don't worsen the pain.

Having pain may limit us physically, and our psychological and emotional tolerance for stress may be lessened. It may be a challenge to adjust to having to give up doing certain things. Affliction with pain and the loss of our abilities to function as fully as we were used to can, indeed, be so traumatic that they take us through all the stages of grief:

- Denial—"No! This can't be happening to me!"

- Bargaining: "Maybe if I [stop doing the things that contributed to getting this pain/get the right treatment/pray], then the pain will go away."

- Suffering the pain: Dealing with the painful sensations; seeking and sorting out options for pain relief; adjusting to the treatments, including side effects; adjusting to not being able to move in particular ways or do certain things; needing to ask for help; adapting to not being able to be there for other people in the same ways as before, and so on.

- Anger: at the pain; at losses of function and compromised quality of life; at ourselves for having contributed (truly or imagined) to the development/appearance of the pain; at others who may have injured or burdened us in some ways that stressed us and left us vulnerable to developing the pain; at other people, such as authorities who did not act in ways to protect us or uncaring people who generically contributed to these circumstances (for example, by polluting the environment, which may have poisoned us, leading to cancer or other painful illnesses); at God for not protecting us from the pain.

- Guilt: over having done or not done things that might have prevented or lessened the pain; feeling that the pain is a cosmic or divine punishment.

- Resolution: Coming to terms with the pain, accepting the limitations it imposes, and learning to live with it.

Any or all of these feelings may surface at any time after starting to suffer pain. They may be clear and unpleasant or subtle and undermining to one's life. As with any other aspect of pain, be it physical or psychological, the more squarely we face our feelings and process them, the easier it is in most cases to go on with life in the best possible ways we can. If we bury our responses to pain and run away from them, they fester and tend to undermine or even poison our lives.

Hillary, a 36-year-old divorced factory employee and single parent of two teenage children, had been a cheerful and pleasant person—until she developed arthritis. The pains she suffered were mainly in her feet and knees, which allowed her to continue working at her sit-down job, with the help of various medications. However, she had great difficulty managing her household chores, which required that she be on her feet a lot.

Even though her son and daughter both pitched in and helped without undue complaints, Hillary became irritable and easily angered, to the point that her relationships with her children began to be strained. Her doctor put her on antidepressants, then on tranquilizers, all to no avail. They only gave her unpleasant side effects.

When she came for a consultation, I suspected that most of her anger was arising from unexpressed disappointment and grief over the limitations she was experiencing due to the arthritis. Hillary had previously enjoyed dancing and walking outdoors in nature or window-shopping with her women friends, and now was frustrated and angry at being unable to enjoy these simple pleasures. She was also angry with herself for being unpleasant to her children and others, but could not control her feelings.

Identifying the underlying issues behind her angers was a help, in and of itself. Using WHEE, Hillary was then able to release these and a pile of other feelings as well. To her surprise, the pains in her feet and knees also improved, and she needed less medication.

Let me be clear here. I am not suggesting that WHEE can totally cure all pains and remove every single distress. However, my experience is that WHEE can certainly help to a significant degree with almost every pain and unpleasant feeling. Most importantly, it can lessen our stress reactions around having the pain and thereby lower our tensions, which otherwise would worsen our pains.

Rewards and Punishments

Once burned, twice shy.

Once pleased, come nigh.

— Anonymous

If we have an enjoyable experience, we want to repeat it; if we suffer a painful experience, we learn to avoid similar situations where we might again be hurt. In psychology this is called *positive and negative reinforcement.* These experiences that shape our lives, teaching us what to pursue and what to avoid, can be perfectly obvious or so subtle that they are completely outside our conscious awareness.

I recall with amusement the story I heard while studying psychology as an undergraduate, about a class that explored positive and negative conditioning on their professor. The students sitting on the right half of the lecture hall nodded their heads and smiled in approval several times during the lecture, while those on the left half shook their heads right to left in disapproval and frowned several times during the lecture. By the end of the hour, the professor was standing on the right side of the hall, talking to the students who were giving him positive reinforcements! He did this without any conscious awareness of what had happened.

Psychological pains are often related to rewards and punishments. People who have suffered the psychological pains of negative experiences will avoid situations that are similar to those in which they were hurt. The child who burns his hand in the kitchen will keep a safe distance from the stove. A person who has had a painful or frightening car crash may become anxious when getting into a car or driving past the scene of the accident. The old suggestion to get back on a horse immediately if you fall off is sound advice. By doing so, you counteract the natural tendency to avoid the painful experience again.

Avoidance reactions to painful situations may be subtle, like the response of the professor in the psychology class. They may also occur early in our lives, being buried and completely forgotten — but still strongly active in motivating us to avoid anything like the painful experiences that we would rather not repeat.

> Pat was an outgoing 32-year-old secretary who lit up any group with her presence. She was popular in the company where she worked, in her church, and loved by her family, but could not maintain a relationship with a man for more than a few weeks. She would often find some reason to break it off, finding fault and blaming her boyfriends for one thing or another. With other lovers, she would be devastated when they left her after brief romances, over what seemed to her to be minor arguments.

> Gradually, it dawned on her that it was rather unlikely that so many men would all be no good. Despite her best efforts, however, Pat could not break the pattern of souring her relationships with men till they split up.

> In the family history she related in her first psychotherapy session, there were very strong hints as to where the problems might have begun. Her father had been alcoholic, a binge drinker who was repeatedly unfaithful to her mother. Pat's parents had divorced when she was 12 and her mother never remarried, remaining bitter and untrusting of men after her unhappy experience in marriage.

> This was a fairly straightforward case, and WHEE was helpful in releasing Pat's buried angers and hurts from having witnessed many arguments and fights between her parents.

It is often the case that we do not see the obvious because we have grown up and lived in the difficult situations that shaped our lives, and they appear perfectly natural to us. Therapists (or family members or friends) may readily help a person to identify such issues because they come to them from outside the situation that generated the negative reactions and led to the burying of the unpleasant feelings.

Pat had been conditioned to mistrust men—both through her direct experiences with her father and through her mother's hurts and angers, which Pat took on as her own views. This had occurred completely outside her awareness, and it took a long time for her to realize that her feelings and behaviors toward men were strongly influenced by her buried inner issues. Her unconscious mind kept telling her she could not trust a man because he was just going to leave her. This mistrust generated emotional responses and behaviors that led Pat to create situations that pushed men away, out of fear that they would leave—in a self-fulfilling prophecy.

Avoiding pains by burying them, running away from them, and then repeating this process with subsequent, similar pains often becomes a self-reinforcing vicious circle. The unconscious mind, programmed in childhood to avoid feeling the pains, continues to find relief from the immediate hurt of new pains by repeating these avoidance maneuvers. The fact that we feel less pain becomes a reinforcement that is similar to the affirming students' smiles. It encourages the unconscious mind to continue these behaviors.

Bereavement is a particularly common psychological pain to be overlooked or avoided. When we feel the pain, sadness, anger, and guilt that are aspects of grief, then all the mechanisms of avoidance detailed above come into play. In addition, in Western society people are encouraged to "be strong" in times of grief and not to display intense emotions in public (whereas in Mediterranean, African, and other cultures, pouring out one's grief in a public manner is encouraged and is the norm.)

Grief over the loss of capabilities and functions due to pain may contribute to making the pains more intense, or to wearing down strength so that the tolerance for pains is lessened. Emotional pain over such losses also may be expressed as a chronic depression.

Buried grief is particularly pernicious in its tendencies to generate, broaden, and perpetuate vicious circles of emotional pain, sadness, anger, and guilt. When landmines of buried grief are present in the unconscious mind, people tiptoe around potential new relationships, avoid anniversary and holiday celebrations, and are put off by shows of any of these feelings in other people—which could release a feared explosion of buried feelings in to consciousness.

> Bruce's dad died when he was 10 years old. Bruce had been very close with him and was devastated. Numerous relatives and several of his teachers thought they were helping when they told him, "Be strong, young man. You have to set a good example for your younger sister and brother, and help your mother now." Bruce bravely held back his tears and pitched in to help his mom at home.

He became a parentified child well before the age when he had the maturity or capabilities to assume such responsibilities. He handled much of the food shopping, supervision of his younger siblings, and chores around the house.

Bruce did well at school and graduated with honors in engineering. He had a job that he liked, which paid well. His boss valued his work highly, as he was extremely careful and never made mistakes.

What appeared at first to be a virtue at work, turned out to be a horrible burden in the rest of his life. Bruce's perfectionism made him a terrible taskmaster to himself. He was constantly monitoring his performance in everything that he did, and excessively critical of any minor mistake or perceived error that others would have ignored or shrugged off. He would obsess over possible errors, over what people would think of him if they noticed his errors, and over excuses he could offer to explain away mistakes.

Needless to say, his perfectionism had also interfered in personal relationships. He had dated numbers of women, but either they ended up not tolerating his perfectionism or he couldn't stand their "messiness."

What brought him to therapy at age 32 was his insomnia. On retiring at night, he would review his day in minute detail, critiquing every error of commission or omission and obsessing over what he could have done differently and better. It was usually one or two in the morning before he fell asleep. Exhausted in the morning, he found his concentration during the day was poorer and poorer and he grew increasingly fearful of making a serious mistake.

While Bruce came in wanting a simple cure for his sleeplessness, it was not hard (to my surprise) to convince him that some detective work to uncover what might be causing his insomnia would be a more thorough approach, and one that would leave him more secure in the permanence of the cure.

Bruce was densely unfamiliar with and not in touch with his feelings. He chose to learn WHEE through a focus on anxieties about his performance at work. The SUDS was an excellent vehicle for Bruce to connect with his inner awareness around intensities and qualities of feelings. At first, he needed many encouragements even to make guesses about what his SUDS might be. Muscle testing was helpful in providing personal feedback and validation of his feelings to himself. This also connected him with his intuitive perceptions and gradually helped him learn to trust them, also.

Muscle testing then helped him trust my suggestion that there might be issues from his past that had sensitized him to making mistakes. Again, I was pleasantly surprised to find Bruce open to exploring within himself in ways that were totally new and unfamiliar. With Bruce's excellent grasp of logic, it was relatively easy to engage him in the detective work required to identify and sort through his life history for possible contributors to his anxieties.

While I could pretty well guess that the heavy load of responsibilities as man of the house in his youth had set him up to worry over failures, this was not the first issue Bruce identified as a contributor to the start of his perfectionism. He recalled a tenth grade teacher who was a stickler for grammar and punctuation. Bruce had written an essay from his heart (not easy for him to do) on the topic, "Taking responsibility for your actions." His teacher, largely ignoring the content, had marked up his paper in red ink over grammar, run-on sentences, missing commas, and the like. Working with WHEE on this issue he had identified for himself, Bruce was pleased to feel the immediate decrease in distress. This lent encouragement as he proceeded with more difficult issues, some of which I suggested, related to his father's absence and his having had to take on a heavy load of responsibilities as a child. Simple *Inner Child* work further facilitated his process.

To his surprise and relief, Bruce was able to fall asleep earlier, without using WHEE directly to address this issue. My intuition was to continue working on his insomnia indirectly.

Though it had not been his primary focus in therapy, Bruce then proceeded to deal with his difficulties in establishing and maintaining relationships with women. It was here that his unresolved grief came out. He had a meta-anxiety about losing close relationships because, from his perspective in childhood, his father had abandoned him when he died. These anxieties were triggered any time he started getting close with women. Releasing the hurt, angers, and guilt associated with the feeling that he had contributed to his father's death by having been a burden to him, Bruce was then able to work on his meta-issues of trusting that he would not be abandoned if he got close with a woman.

Sorting out all of these issues was also a cure for Bruce's insomnia. He found that the habit of worrying into sleeplessness would occasionally return when he was stressed. At those times he dealt with it successfully, using WHEE directly to fall asleep.

I cannot count the times I have seen unresolved grief fester for years until an opportunity arose for the unconscious to release these buried feelings. The landmine of buried, unexpressed bereavement can be triggered by personal life events, media, anniversaries, and so forth, or can arise spontaneously—either gradually or suddenly—for no apparent reason. The effects of unexpressed grief are often subtle and pernicious, as was the case in Bruce's life.

Commonly overlooked causes for bereavement include miscarriages and abortions. Women who experience these are often expected to pick themselves up and move on with life, with no processing or clearing of their feelings.

Another common loss is that of a pet. Dogs, cats, and other animals become family members. They are loved and offer their unconditional love, yet their loss may be minimized because they are not human. Such loss, however, may be all the more intense because in many cases the people with whom the pets lived have had to make a decision about ending their suffering rather than letting them live in pain and discomfort. This may add layers of guilt and hurt to the bereavement.

Bereavement is a factor that may be missed in some cases in therapy, particularly when therapists have not cleared their own buried grief reactions. Another way that buried grief may be missed is through focusing primarily on the presenting symptoms and not doing a wholistic, thorough housecleaning.

Having experienced the pain of bereavement, a person will deepen their resonations with the suffering of others and more readily come to a place of compassion.

Before you know kindness as the deepest thing inside,
you must know sorrow
as the other deepest thing.
You must wake up with sorrow.
You must speak to it till your voice
catches the thread of all sorrows
and you see the size of the cloth.

Then it is only kindness that makes sense anymore,
only kindness that ties your shoes
and sends you out into the day
to mail letters and purchase bread,
only kindness that raises its head
from the crowd of the world to say
it is I you have been looking for,
and then goes with you everywhere
like a shadow or a friend.

— Naomi Shihab Nye

Physical pains often have strong components of learned responses, too. These responses become associated with tension in the context of an original emotional trauma. Thereafter, we may experience the same tensing-up response in similarly stressful situations. A case of this kind was presented to me when a young woman sought my help with a personal problem.

Kate was a vivacious young college student who suffered from frequent, horrendous headaches. She thought these were just something she had to bear, as her mother and sister also had bad headaches and Kate believed these simply ran in her family through their genes.

Kate came for therapy when she began to notice that many of her headaches started when she was interacting with men, particularly with handsome men. Her headaches came on not just in dating situations, but also with men in her classes and in the office where she worked part-time.

In reviewing her headache history in her initial psychotherapy session, Kate recalled clearly that her first headache had occurred when she was dating a boy in high school whom she found very attractive. He was giving clear indications that he wanted to have sex, which went against Kate's strict religious upbringing. She developed such a severe headache that they cut their date short.

From that time onward, Kate suffered headaches whenever she was in the presence of a man who appeared to be getting close to her. With little prompting, she was able to see that headaches in these situations were a bad habit that she had developed. (She also had headaches in other situations, but we left those to be dealt with at a later time.)

These sorts of symptoms, like the reaction of the professor to the students' smiles and frowns, are called *reinforced responses*. When we do something that is rewarded, we tend to do it again; when it is punished, we tend to do it less often. The rewards, the learned lessons, and the repetitions are often completely unconscious. Kate's unconscious mind got her out of her conflict between her sexual responsiveness and her strict upbringing through the painful headaches that gave her an "out" from those situations that she did not know how to resolve.

Using WHEE, Kate was able within 45 minutes to release her anxieties about relating to men sexually. Part of the work was also to release her anxieties about behaving inappropriately if she allowed herself to feel her sexual feelings. She quickly came to see that she could use good judgment and common sense without holding onto the beliefs about retribution in Hell and other intense religious fears that had plagued her.

In two brief telephone follow-up sessions, Kate dealt with other issues that had hitched themselves to her tendencies to have headaches, including dealing with other anxieties and fears, and expressing anger.

Many sorts of issues can make us emotionally or psychologically uptight, which can then make our body uptight, creating various pains.

The initial phase of a WHEE session therefore involves detective work to clarify who did what, when, and with what rewards or consequences in the past, resulting in vicious circles of anxiety → worry → tension → pain → more anxiety.

Often, we are so used to our ways of responding that we don't see the patterns or connections behind our pains. A therapist can help us identify how we were reinforced to respond with pain and suggest helpful ways to address the patterns. This is not to say we can't do this ourselves, but that the therapist can save us a lot of time and point out issues and ways of dealing with them that we might never notice or think about.

Like Kate, we may feel conflicted between our conscience and our desires over many types of issues. Pain can divert us away from our tensions. This may happen over issues such as:

- Being unhappy in a work situation but feeling we must stick it out and not be a "quitter."

- Lacking confidence in our abilities but feeling we should push ourselves to do something difficult.

- Having habits (such as eating, smoking, drinking, or drug abuse) and finding ourselves unable to stop our cravings or change our behaviors.

Yet another way that pain may become a stronger and more persistent visitor in our lives is through the rewards we get from having the pains. When other people are more attentive to us, or when the pains provide excuses for not having to do things we would rather avoid (but hesitated to assert ourselves to deal with directly), this can become a powerful reinforcer. Again, just like with the professor, this can be a totally unconscious process.

Common ways we may get caught in reinforced pain responses include:

- A chance injury or illness is painful. Well-meaning family and friends are more solicitous and helpful than usual.

- Someone in our family, often a parent or older sibling, has pains and gets attention or special consideration because of their distress.

- We see an example of rewarded pain in a film or on TV.

In these situations, our unconscious mind may say, "Here's a way to get more caring, help or attention." So, our body helps us by recreating the pain when we're feeling stressed or needy.

Sometimes, pain serves multiple functions. Part of Kate's pain pattern was that she felt so bad about her sexual feelings that some unconscious part of her believed she deserved to be punished for them. Thus, pain not only got her out of her situation of forbidden temptations, it also punished her for her perceived transgressions of taboos from her religious upbringing.[3]

When new pains arise in our lives, both physical and emotional, they may stir the pot of memories and help us to release old issues like Pat's, which were thoroughly buried and completely forgotten. Each new experience of pain is thus an invitation and opportunity for making a shift toward better ways of handling both the new and the old pains. Eventually, we may even come to the point that we totally release the child habits of burying pains.

At times, looking back on experiences like these, it appears that our unconscious mind may set us up with pains as a way to finally release the buried hurts it has been carrying. I have worked with people who developed migraines, irritable bowel syndrome, backaches, fibromyalgia, and other problems that ended up being extremely helpful to them in the long run in such ways.[4]

How We Are Programmed to Get in Trouble

People are taught that pain is evil and dangerous. How can they deal with love if they're afraid to feel? Pain is meant to wake us up. People try to hide their pain. But they're wrong. Pain is something to carry, like a radio. You feel your strength in the experience of pain. It's all in how you carry it. That's what matters. Pain is a feeling. Your feelings are a part of you. Your own reality. If you feel ashamed of them, and hide them, you're letting society destroy your reality. You should stand up for your right to feel your pain.

—Jim Morrison

[3] Dealing with self-rewarding pain can be a challenge. This topic is discussed in detail in Chapter 4.
[4] For more on such workings of the unconscious mind, see Chapter 5. (On litigation as a factor in pain see Chapter 8.)

A natural question to ask is, "Why do we get ourselves in trouble and lock ourselves into vicious circles?"

Our problems begin when we all make the silly mistake of letting a little child program our lifetime computer. Dr. Judith Swack calls this "baby logic." As children, we often cannot understand the reasons for painful or frightening situations. Children cannot change their unpleasant circumstances, cannot leave, cannot fire or exchange their parents. We are stuck in unhappiness, and do not even have a full concept of time to know that a painful experience will eventually end. A young infant who is crying in her crib because she is hungry has no way to know that her hunger pangs will ever be relieved or that she will ever feel comforted again.

In such situations, it is very helpful for us to run away from the hurt or to forget it, burying the feelings outside of conscious awareness. As children, this is a good choice for dealing with pain and suffering, since we cannot avoid it. Our unconscious mind then gets used to protecting us from the distress of these hurts by keeping them firmly locked away so that we cannot sense them and do not suffer from them.

Our buried feeling memories are stored in unconscious parts of the right side of the brain. The right brain puts a sign on the locked closet saying, "Keep Away!!" It then says to the left brain, where our conscious mind resides, "We don't want to know about this, do we?" And the left brain says, "No, let's stay away from those painful memories and feelings." So we pretend to ourselves that they aren't there.

While this system works well to protect us as children from fears and pains, it soon becomes the default for our lifetime "computer guidance" programs. As we get older, these programs become outmoded. We acquire greater capacities to cope with life and deal with problems in more mature ways. However, the unconscious mind remains afraid of the buried feelings locked away in its closets. It believes that the original, buried fears and hurts might still overwhelm us with all the intensity of our original reactions from the time when we buried them. The unconscious mind, still working according to the child programs, doesn't know that we can handle these feelings better as adults. For example: The right brain puts a memo in fine print under the Keep Away sign on the closet where fears from our parents' arguments are buried, saying, "Stay away from anything like an argument or angry people." We may then end up cutting ourselves off from experiences and relationships that otherwise might have been much better tolerated as adults, such as avoiding people with loud voices or people who resemble our parents in other ways.

> *Numbing the pain for a while will make it worse*
> *when you finally feel it.*
>
> —J. K. Rowling

If we encounter something in our current life that rattles the skeletons in the closets of our unconscious mind, it is possible that the door to frightening memories could pop open a crack, and we might feel some of the original, buried feelings. This is why we sometimes over-react when a person in our current life reminds us of someone who frightened or hurt us in the past.

For example, I had a lot of anger toward my mother as a child, but buried it because she was a single parent and I did not feel safe expressing it, nor did I find other outlets for these angers. For years, I was easily angered by authority figures, particularly aggressive women.

In another example, we might have buried anxieties and fears from when we were jealous of a brother or sister. As adults, if we encounter someone who is like our sibling, they may make us very uncomfortable—completely out of proportion to what is happening in the present; but we respond with unwarranted hurt or anger because of the memories and feelings that are stirred in the closets holding our memories.

As adults, our unconscious resists releasing these emotions buried in the caverns of our being—even when we are no longer in the painful situations that caused them and are clearly in a better position to deal with them. Our child programs persist and prevail: "Don't let these feelings out! They are dangerous and painful and you won't know what to do with them."

These childhood programs operate in general as well as in specific ways. As adults, we continue to stuff uncomfortable feelings inside, shutting the door behind them. Often, rather than letting out the displaced angers that are generated by situations in the present that resonate with the past, we stuff more unpleasant feelings in our inner filing cabinets.

While self-healing techniques and various therapies can help to release some of these well-hidden traumas, our inner programs resist such efforts. Often, it is only when the emotional pus from past hurts festers to the point of serious physical and emotional pain that we even begin to become aware that something distressing is inside us.

Many of us spend our whole lives running from feeling with the mistaken belief that you cannot bear the pain. But you have already borne the pain. What you have not done is feel all you are beyond the pain.

—Saint Bartholomew

Physical pain may thus be a signal from our unconscious, saying that our file drawers are so full that it is becoming a burden to keep the conscious mind from feeling these buried hurts and angers.

Much of your pain is self-chosen.

It is the bitter potion by which the physician within you heals your sick self.

Therefore trust the physician, and drink his remedy in silence and tranquility:

For his hand, though heavy and hard, is guided by the tender hand of the Unseen,

And the cup he brings, though it burn your lips, has been fashioned of the clay which the Potter has moistened with His own sacred tears.

—Khalil Gibran

One very literal way in which our mind and body get us into trouble is with eating problems. These are complex and, as anyone who has struggled with weight control will testify, can be very challenging to address. I discuss this here because being overweight commonly represents a combination of psychological factors at work and can contribute to pains of many origins.

Al was a 35-year-old accountant who suffered severe backaches over several years. He was carrying 320 pounds on a body that was only 5' 7" tall—clearly more than was healthy.

Al readily admitted to having difficulties controlling his eating. He enjoyed eating, often having second or even third portions of foods he particularly liked. He also engaged in comfort eating, particularly when stressed. Holidays and other celebrations and the months before taxes were due were times when he was most unhappy with himself about his overeating.

His worsening backaches were what brought Al for help with WHEE. Due to their multiple side effects, he had found no pain medicine with which he was comfortable. He was hoping that WHEE would allow him at least to suffer less, if not to completely free him from the misery he experienced in getting out of a chair, standing in line at the bank or supermarket, walking about, and in most other activities.

As part of my complete review of his life history, we discussed his weight issues. He had found no diets, weight control support groups, or other therapies that helped more than briefly before he returned to overeating and gave up the treatments in frustration and disgust.

Al was surprised when I suggested that the first thing he should do was to eat as he normally did, but when I instructed him in journaling he began to understand what was going on and what he was feeling whenever he ate more than he knew was good for him.

He returned the next week with a prioritized list, the worst eating-inducing problem at the top and the least at the bottom. His highest ranked item was stress. WHEE worked wonders on this for about two weeks, to his great delight. Whenever he was stressed and feeling hungry, he reduced the SUDS for the stress and his hunger abated. However, the next week Al was back, disappointed and feeling that WHEE would be just another method to add to his list of failures. He had had several serious problems at work, his stress levels were not responding to WHEE, and his appetite was again out of control.

I had alerted Al that this might happen, and that dealing with his eating habits was likely to be something of a roller-coaster ride. This helped him cope with his initial disappointment and discouragement when his first spurt of improvement did not turn into a permanent resolution of his eating difficulties.

We explored for meta-feelings and meta-beliefs that might be getting in the way of his releasing. In dialogue with his inner, critical parent, he found that he was afraid he would "lose his edge of alertness" if he let go of his anxieties completely. He was able to reach a compromise with his Inner Parent that they could release a little more of the anxiety at a time, observing carefully for any signs of his becoming careless in his accounting work before letting go any further.

Al also searched in the file drawers of his memories from childhood for anything related to this current meta-anxiety. He found memories of his mother being extremely critical of his father and of him whenever they made mistakes, particularly when they forgot things. This carried a level-8 SUDS, with accompanying tightness in his throat and stomach. Connecting with his Inner Child, Al was able to release this rapidly, installing a replacement affirmation of "I can be gentle with myself when I make mistakes that aren't work related."

In the following week, Al was pleased to find that he was able to control his eating even better than in the first two weeks. At his next session, he reported he was much more optimistic than he had been in a long time about dealing with his overeating.

Al's experience is a good example of addressing pain with wholistic approaches. When Al came to therapy for his back pain, he never imagined we'd be considering his mother being critical of his father. Yet this was one of the causes behind his internalized critical parent, which was contributing to much of his comfort eating.

You might have noticed I did not encourage Al to use WHEE for his backaches in this early phase of treatment. While there was every reason to expect WHEE would work well for his pain, it would not have been in his best interests to remove this motivating reminder from his unconscious about needing to attend to the weight that was adding a constant to his back. If Al did not identify and deal with the underlying causes behind his overeating, WHEE would just become another on his long list of failed, discarded therapies.

Working bit by bit on the issues that Al identified which led him to overeat, he was able to reduce weight for the first time in many years.

This was an excellent preparation in several respects for his then using the WHEE directly for his pain.

How the Unconscious Speaks to Us

If you are visited by pain, examine your conduct.

—Talmud

Programmed by a child, the unconscious mind continues to think, feel, and act like a child. When it wants relief from discomfort, tensions, worries, fears, or angers, it wants it *now!* Most of the time, we are not aware of this inner distress. In some cases, though, the distress becomes severe and the unconscious gets more and more upset, and then seeks ways to get our attention for relief.

Unconscious distress may build up in two ways. First, there may be repeated traumas over time that fill the inner filing cabinets, garbage cans, and caves to overflowing. Second, as we mature, our unconscious begins to realize that it might be able to explore new and better ways of handling problems. In either case, the unconscious then seeks to unburden itself of the job of keeping the lid tightly shut on our awareness of these buried feelings.

As our unconscious becomes increasingly ready to let go of old hurts, the conscious mind may not understand that it is now okay to recall and feel the buried hurts. When that happens, the unconscious starts to clamor for their release. We may become uneasy or anxious in situations where more of the same negative feelings are experienced and then stashed away by the unconscious, adding to the pressures for release. If we don't attend to these gentler alerts and calls for help through anxieties, our unconscious turns up the volume. We may have dreams or nightmares that call our attention to these issues. If we still do not respond, the unconscious may demand our attention through physical symptoms, the most common of which is pain.

I developed a moderately strong, aching, squeezing pain in my chest as I was speaking on the phone. On the other end of the line was "Joan," a woman with whom I had had an intense relationship that did not hold us together strongly enough to navigate the stormy waters and reefs of divergent personal beliefs, preferences, and lifestyles. We were clearing the air of residual feelings and clarifying some of our misunderstandings so that we could return to being friends and colleagues.

The pain was strong enough to worry me—almost enough to make it difficult to breathe. I had no history of heart disease, but this is no guarantee of not having a heart attack. The symptoms fit that pattern.

However, the timing of the pain was too clearly punctuating the emotional heartache I was feeling with my deep disappointment over our breakup. Not feeling that it was appropriate to process this during our conversation for healing hurts, angers and misunderstandings, farewells to intimacy, and movement back toward our earlier modes of relating, I did some quiet, deep breathing exercises as we wound down the conversation and said our goodbyes.

I then went into a quiet, meditative, inward place of peace, where I could invite my pain to speak to me. As I have done this many times before, I rapidly received a number of deeply felt responses.

First, there was my heartache—the deep sadness and hurt of disappointment in the breakup of my relationship with Joan. Then came anger at her and at myself, for things said and unsaid, done and held back from doing. Then more sadness. After crying my heart out over parting with Joan, the pain diminished by about two thirds.

From experience, I know that this sort of deep pain usually sits in the same file drawer with earlier, similar pains. I invited my Inner Child to release any similar pains, with their associated memories. Again, I felt a flood of hurt and anger over feeling abandoned by each of my parents. My mother was unable to be present for me in ways I felt I wanted and needed as a child, and my father was physically absent.

I used WHEE to clear these layers of childhood feelings and issues, and after that, to release more layers of the recent feelings and issues with Joan. When I finished, my pain was completely cleared.

While I may well have used WHEE to help me clear my feelings arising from the current issues of the terminated relationship, I might not have looked for the earlier feelings of rejection and hurt—if my unconscious had not created that pain in my chest. This pain alerted me that there might be issues much deeper than the current disappointment and hurt that were sitting in that inner file drawer, ready for release and asking me to clear them.

In this case, the pain around my heart spoke clearly of its origins: the heartaches of current and past feelings around not being wanted. I have seen pains in the throat or stomach from swallowing down feelings; pains in the neck or head from irritations that people complain are "a pain in the neck" or "a big headache"; and many, many other metaphoric pains.[5]

In other instances, it may not be obvious why the unconscious mind chooses particular symptoms to draw our attention to specific inner issues it wants us to address. Usually, this is more like a pipe leaking corrosive, negative feelings rather than a volcano that is spewing out fire and brimstone—although major eruptions of unconscious distress are also possible.

Another lesson to take away from this experience is that our relationships often bring out buried feelings that we have not identified on our own. Our unconscious mind has an uncanny ability to pick exactly the right partner who will trigger those buried hurts that we most need to release, but that we are most reluctant or unable to identify on our own.

The Inner Child

> *A torn jacket is soon mended;*
> *but hard words bruise the heart of a child.*
>
> —Henry Wadsworth Longfellow

Each of us has a part of ourselves that remains a child throughout our lifetime. This is the part that wants to be fully and totally accepted, loved, and nurtured; to be guided by competent adults to learn ways of behaving that are acceptable; and to be unfettered by what it feels are

---

[5] For a more complete list of metaphoric pains, see *Healing Research, Volume 2.*

unjust restrictions on its freedom by others' wishes, wills, and actions. Sigmund Freud called this the *id*; Eric Berne relabeled it the *Child*.

At various times in our day, in response to whatever may happen in our lives, our Inner Child may be fun-loving and playful, ready to enjoy the pleasures of life. He may be sensitive and petulant, hurt by experienced or perceived rebuffs or slights. She may be rebellious and oppositional, angrily insisting on her way or no way.

Even though we may be well past our childhood years, our Inner Child persists as a strongly felt presence—though mostly this is very much outside our conscious awareness. In addition to patterns of beliefs and behaviors, our Inner Child retains factual and feeling memories of childhood experiences. Whatever we experienced that left a major impression will remain as part of our Inner Child.

The childhood process of avoiding and burying painful feelings and memories was discussed above. Our Inner Child continues to function with the rules it developed in childhood. However, as adults we are able to negotiate with our Inner Child and can help her or him to release some of the old, buried hurts, angers, and fears, as well as to change the Inner Child's rules about dealing with new and buried feelings and memories. Such releases are illustrated in my own experience and in the example of Al, above.

The Inner Child releases pains and other problems much more readily and easily than the adult. It appears that the Inner Child who persists inside us is truly a child in mental processes as well as in memories and childish responses to situations. Thus, accessing our Inner Child when the SUDS or SUSS is not moving provides us with another tool for handling resistances.

Dialoguing with Our Inner Child

Never a lip is curved with pain that can't be kissed into smiles again.

—Bret Harte

It is surprising how readily available our Inner Child may be. We will often find a full and open response to a simple invitation to speak—sometimes with much more information than we might have expected. The experience I shared above about processing my feelings following the breakup of a relationship shows how this can happen. Here is another example:

> At a workshop with 400 people, Michelle volunteered to use WHEE in front of the audience for relief of shoulder pains. Prior to the demonstration, this woman who appeared to be in her late fifties clarified that she had not been able to lift her arms above shoulder height for several years. She was also suffering from pains during the night that interrupted her sleep.
>
> When she came up for the demonstration, she added that she also had back and hip pains that she had not disclosed to me earlier. Working on all of the current pains combined produced no relief in any of them over a period of ten minutes. This is unusual for WHEE, unless there are other issues associated with the pains. (I must admit, I was a bit anxious that the demonstration would not be an advertisement for benefits of WHEE, and thinking I might well use it for my own stress!)
>
> I invited her to focus just on her initial complaint of shoulder pains, and to connect with her Inner Child to explore the origins of the pains. She readily recalled the pains beginning when she was emotionally abused by her father in childhood. When she included these memories in using WHEE, she experienced a dramatic lessening of her shoulder pains.

My personal experience, and that of countless people I have worked with, is that when we connect with the Inner Child we release our feelings and issues with WHEE in the same manner that a child would respond. In the above example, Michelle had repeatedly buried her feelings of fear, hurt, and anger during childhood. The repetitions placed extra-strong locks on the doors of her inner filing cabinets. Her unconscious mind, however, tightened up her back muscles till they hurt. Michelle learned to live with these pains, not understanding their origins and not knowing what to do about them.

When she grew up and her father passed on, Michelle's unconscious mind knew that there was no further danger and no real reason to keep carrying all of those buried feelings. At the same time, the habits of keeping the feelings firmly locked away from conscious awareness were very strong. It would appear that her unconscious mind created the shoulder pains to invite Michelle to do the clearing she did with WHEE.

I've been pleased to find that many people who have had no prior experience of connecting with their Inner Child are able to do so quickly, easily, deeply, and with excellent results.

Alice, a woman in her mid-fifties, spoke with me on the phone about a business matter totally unrelated to WHEE. She mentioned that her left ankle had been acting up, feeling tight and not as stable as the other one. I offered to introduce her to WHEE and she readily agreed.

Dialoguing with her ankle, she sensed immediately that a current conflict in her life was making her uptight and that this was probably reactivating residuals of an injury that had occurred at age 10, with several subsequent re-injuries. Alice laughed as she realized that when she was stressed, she also was often heard to say, "I'm up to my ankles in snakes!"

Alice started using WHEE, tapping her eyebrows and saying, "Even though I feel distressed, concerned, fearful, protective and confused, when I think about this unpleasant situation and the tightness in my ankle, I still love and accept myself, wholly and completely." She then added that she also felt love when she focused on the situation. In one round of WHEE, her tension went from a level 10 to a 4. Adding to her initial counteracting affirmation, "and the Infinite Source loves and accepts me, wholly and completely and unconditionally" as she tapped a second time, her SUDS level went down to zero. She also remarked that there was a palpably stronger effect with the addition of the Infinite Source to the counteracting affirmation.

Having heard that Alice's ankle had been injured at age 10, I asked her what recollections and feelings she had from that experience. She could not come up with any memories or emotions related to the incident. However, when she went back in her memory to being 10-year-old Alice, she immediately recalled being pushed by some bullies when she was tobogganing, ending up flipping the toboggan and fracturing her ankle. The only strong feeling she felt with this long-buried memory was betrayal, and this was at a level 15 (on a scale of 10). Alice was able to clear this feeling in several rounds of WHEE.

She could immediately see that betrayal was also a feeling that had been stirred in her current situation. Having cleared the memories and feelings from age 10, she felt no further need to clear anything around the tightness in her ankle, from the current situation or any earlier time in her life.

The positive statement Alice chose to install was, "Betrayal is only in the moment. It doesn't reflect on me as a person, and I can stay in a place of love." This was already at a strongly positive level of 10 and needed no enhancing with WHEE.

In other instances, people find that the Inner Child is distrustful and negotiations are more difficult. They have to promise that they will continue to nurture the needs of their Inner Child—and make good on their promises—before they are able to get his cooperation in exploring and releasing old hurts. This can be quite challenging and may require skilled guidance from a therapist. Once the Inner Child comes on board, however, progress is usually rapid.

Another major way in which we can help ourselves is in learning to give love to our Inner Child, particularly when we experienced neglect or abuse in our childhood. Conversely, the Inner Child may take a while to learn to accept the love we are offering him or her. This can be a challenge from both sides, because the adult may have difficulty giving the Inner Child love at the same time that the Inner Child has a hard time accepting it. In my personal work with my Inner Child, hugging a teddy bear while nurturing my Inner Child has been very helpful. Persistence does pay off! When our Inner Child can accept our love, then we as adults are much better able to anticipate and accept love from others.

Vicious Circles that Lock In Our Pain

The trick is not how much pain you feel, but how much joy you feel. Any idiot can feel pain. Life is full of excuses to feel pain, excuses not to live, excuses, excuses, excuses.

—Erica Jong

Once we are experiencing pain, it is very easy to get caught up in various vicious circles that keep us in pain. A common way we may drift into a vicious circle is through tension. Tense muscles will ultimately start to complain by hurting. Backaches and headaches are common results of stress, but other muscles can also spasm and ache. Once we feel the pain, a vicious circle is initiated: pain → emotional tension → anxiety → more muscle tension → spasm → increased pain → increased tension and anxiety, and so on.

Similar muscle spasms from stresses and tensions produce a narrowing of the airways in the bronchioles, the smaller tubes in our lungs, bringing on asthmatic attacks. Tension in arteries throughout our body results in elevated blood pressure, while spasms in arteries of our heart cause angina (heart pain from insufficient blood supply) and in muscles along the skull producing migraines. Spasms in the muscles of our gut contribute to irritable bowel syndrome and colitis. Excessive gastric acid secretion leads to heartburn and worsening ulcers...and the list of other such disorders goes on.

Subtler and more insidious changes in the immune system may also occur due to chronic tensions. White cells and antibodies are less effective in protecting the health of people who are under stress. This may contribute to the development of infections, and may increase our susceptibility to serious illnesses such as AIDS and cancer.

Psychological vicious circles also lock in our pain. Starting in childhood, we bury our hurts and spend much of our lives running away from them. Since this is a successful maneuver, helping us avoid feeling the original pain or feeling the memories of the pain, we continue to do so, like the drunk who snapped his fingers to scare away the pink elephants. When someone pointed out that there were no pink elephants around, he replied, "See! It works!"

It is easy to fall into the habit patterns of continuing to bury current hurts rather than dealing with them. These contribute to our being anxious and tense, which can then contribute to whatever physical pains we have. Our childhood anxieties and fears are the locks on the file drawers where our pains are buried. Until we address these fears, we may be unable to release the hurts.[6]

---

[6] We will explore how to do this in Chapter 3, in the section on meta-anxieties.

Secondary Gain

Secondary gain can also initiate cycles that maintain and per-petuate pain and other symptoms. Pain may be useful, consciously or unconsciously, in some situations—despite the fact that it causes us discomfort and we consciously wish to be rid of it. For example, pain can provide an acceptable excuse for not attending a social event that might be stressful, for avoiding unwanted sexual relations, for not going to work, or for side-stepping other unpleasant obligations or demands. Conversely, a symptom may bring us caring responses from family and friends, and greater closeness—in relationships where we hesitate to ask for such attention, or where others hesitate to offer it.

The unconscious mind, searching for the most immediate way to relieve our anxieties, might thus help us avoid facing stressful situa-tions by perpetuating or even aggravating present pains of any cause. A chronic headache may flare up conveniently (though unconsciously) when my mother-in-law phones to invite me to dinner. Secondary gain may then reinforce the pain-tension-spasm cycle when this pattern recurs in other situations as well. As Sherwood Anderson noted, "The sick man is more than half a rascal. He may only be sick because he hasn't the courage to clean house."

Transactional Analysis

Wisdom is knowing what to do next; virtue is doing it.

—David Starr Jordan

Eric Berne's simplified language of Transactional Analysis (TA) for psychoanalytic understandings of how people tick can be enormously helpful when combined with WHEE. Berne observed that everyone (regardless of our age) has three basic *ego states*: the inner *Parent, Adult,* and *Child.* (See Figure 1.)

Our inner Parent tells us what we should and shouldn't do. This is the part that was programmed by our own parents, schoolteach-ers, religious teachers, and the authorities of our broader society. This Parent can speak with a supportive voice or a critical tone. We often become aware of this part as a problem when we are "shoulding" on ourselves.

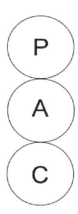

Figure 1. TA ego states.

The Inner Adult computes the logical likelihood of our succeeding in getting what we want in life (like Mr. Spock in *Star Treck*), taking into account our inner and outer awareness.

And the Inner Child wants to be able to express its feelings and have what it wants when it wants it. Our Inner Child may express itself in a simple, *natural*, unfettered way; it may *adapt* its expressions of feelings in order to be accepted or, at least, not rejected; or it may *rebel* in order to get its own way in the face of opposition or criticism.

I find that there is an additional aspect to the Inner Child, the *pain body*, as described by Eckhart Tolle.[7] This is the hurt child that responds with pain, fear and anger when the child feels he or she is mistreated, and can lash out in anger when we are feeling distressed as adults, or even generate anger and pain.

TA is an extremely helpful map for self-healing. If you find yourself in conflict with other people and you listen to how they are speaking and to how you are thinking, feeling, and speaking, you may very quickly identify why there is friction between you.

> Louise asked her teenage daughter, "When are you going to clean up your room?" Louise's conscious intent was simply to know when the floor would be clear so that she could vacuum it. Tammy responded angrily, "Why are you always nagging and criticizing

---

[7] The pain body is discussed further in Chapter 6.

me?" Louise was surprised to hear her so upset, when she was asking a simple question and looking for a factual answer.

When we re-enacted the encounter in a family counseling session, it became clear that while Louise's words were coming from her Adult ego state, her tone of voice had a distinct edge of Critical Parent in it (because she had actually asked Tammy this question more than just once before). Tammy was responding to her mother's Critical Parent tone rather than to her factual, Adult message.

It is extremely common to find that you and others respond more to the feeling tone of a message than to its content. So if you get an unexpected response, you might ask yourself, "What feeling tones are being expressed here?" This may rapidly help you understand where you are coming from when you get into conflicts, especially when these seem illogical relative to the content of your verbal exchanges.

The second helpful aspect to this map is that it immediately suggests alternatives to the conflict-ridden exchanges. You could choose to change your tone of voice and feeling focus to that of the Supportive Parent. This might get a better response: "I know this isn't your favorite of all things to do on a Saturday morning, but I need to vacuum and I'd really appreciate your help in getting the house cleaned." Or you might shift to Adult (with a neutral tone), "When you've cleaned your room, we can go out shopping for your school clothes;" or speak from your own Child ego state, "I hate to have to do the cleaning as much as you do, but if we get it done quickly and without fuss we can both have the rest of the day to enjoy ourselves."

All of these observations are easy to make from our calm states of emotions and mind when we are not in the midst of a stressful or distressing situation. Our problems may be harder to deal with when we are in the midst of outer confrontations and mixed responses from our inner ego states. When we look back on a situation and are unhappy with the responses we gave, we can identify the negative thoughts and feelings we experienced and use WHEE to clear them. Then, we can install replacement positives for the negatives we released. Once we are familiar with this process, we can use it in the actual situation.

Sol returned from work at a construction company, tired and frustrated about problems with his boss and with several co-workers over a rushed repair job that had not gone well. Molly, his wife, had been waiting all afternoon for his return, eager for his help in preparation for their dinner party that evening. Among other tasks needing his assistance, she could not manage to take down some dishes herself from the top of a kitchen cabinet because of her chronic back pain.

Sol had been looking forward to a refreshing shower and a little chill-out in front of the TV prior to the dinner. He caught his Inner Child wanting to react from a place of tiredness and anger. Having been to counseling over his hot temper, he chose to excuse himself to take a quick time out to calm down before responding to Molly. Using WHEE, he was able to release most of his feelings of frustration and anger from work. He could then respond to Molly from a place of Supportive Parent and Natural Child.

Sol illustrates some of the ways WHEE can be helpful to family members and caregivers working with people who have pain. We want to be there to help, but sometimes feel our own needs may be neglected or set aside because the person in pain is suffering. By releasing the frustrations that can introduce negative feelings into our interactions, we are freed up to respond from a more healing space.

I will refer to TA in several other sections as a very helpful framework for applying WHEE.

Psychological Pain

*Pain (any pain—emotional, physical, mental) has a message....
Once we get the pain's message, and follow its advice, the pain goes
away.*

— Peter McWilliams

Stress and distress are often painful. This is particularly true with major traumatic experiences such as sexual abuse or rape; or personally suffering or observing someone else experiencing a serious injury. These traumas can produce reactions so severe that people have difficulties functioning normally in their lives. They may become overly emotional with minimal stress, easily angered, or phobic about situations and relationships similar to the original traumas. They may re-enact the trauma in various ways, have low self-esteem, difficulties concentrating and sleeping, nightmares, headaches, backaches, and other symptoms. This is called post-traumatic stress disorder (PTSD) and may be so severe as to be incapacitating or may even lead to suicide. This is a particularly painful problem with war veterans, as the US Veterans' Administration Hospitals have not been very responsive to these issues.

I digress a little here to address another issue with PTSD. I have seen many people overeat as one of their unconscious ways of dealing with severe stress reactions, particularly sexual traumas. This serves a variety of defensive functions. Comfort eating can become a substitute gratification for avoided social relationships, guilt, and self-blame (common in victims of abuse), frustrations with emotional liability and temper outbursts, and low self-esteem. By putting on weight, people with PTSD may also feel they are "armored" against physical intrusions and less likely to attract sexual attentions.

The overeating may become a serious issue when one's muscles, bones, and joints start to complain of the load being carried—with backaches or pains in knees and hips, elevated blood pressure, heart strain, diabetes, or other metabolic fallout from being overweight. WHEE can help with all of these secondary problems through stress and pain reductions, but is most important to use for dealing with the overeating that underlies the secondary problems.

Overeating is actually an issue of cravings and may take on the proportions of an addiction. Eating is one of the most difficult of cravings/addictions to deal with because one can't stop completely, and because there are constant exposures to temptations. WHEE works well and quickly, as mentioned, for reducing and eliminating cravings directly. Addressing the underlying issues behind the cravings for food is a matter for long-term therapy. WHEE is enormously helpful here, too, in addressing issues of the underlying traumas, self-image, self-confidence, social problems, and more.

I return now to further issues surrounding PTSD. Memories of traumas may be triggered, altogether unexpectedly, by life circumstances that resonate with the original distress. Coming out of the freezer chest of trauma and warming into an intimate relationship is a common such trigger. Being injured or undergoing medical examinations or procedures that touch upon body parts that were traumatized, even during a massage, is another common stimulus to rousing traumatic memories.

Sometimes stresses that seem minor in relation to one's life as a whole may nevertheless have a major traumatic impact. The resultant PTSD can be much more subtle, with covert and delayed reactions. Children's behaviors often change drastically in response to such traumas. They may become uncharacteristically silent or overemotional, have a major drop in academic performance, and withdraw from social interactions and relationships. It also is not uncommon for memories of childhood physical, emotional, or sexual abuse to be buried and forgotten for many years.

Here are two such examples:

Christie was criticized severely in front of the whole class by her fourth grade teacher for making several errors in reciting a poem that had been assigned as homework. Christie had always been a little shy in public speaking, which probably contributed to her poor poetry recitation. This experience was very traumatic for her and imprinted Christie with the belief that she was terrible at public speaking, a belief that persisted and grew worse through her life. She was perfectly comfortable speaking in front of her immediate family and with two to three close friends, but her mind went blank in front of any larger group.

* * *

Norman was horrified to walk into a university cafeteria and see his girlfriend holding hands with his best friend. He broke off the relationship in great distress. Following this experience, he developed a distrust of women and major doubts about his ability to be attractive to them. He remained single for many years, despite being a personable, attractive young man.

Such relatively minor experiences can scar a person for years, sometimes for life. The childhood habits of keeping these memories buried and then running away from them may be effective as far as helping to not suffer the agonies of buried past pains, but this often generates great distress and pain in the present.

Others who may suffer are caregivers and emergency service workers, who may experience secondary PTSD in the course of observing or treating people who are suffering from pain and PTSD. In some cases caregivers may uncover previously unrecognized traumatic events in their own lives through the triggers of treating traumatized people.

Often, these psychological pains are associated with tensions in the body that end up causing physical pain. Frozen shoulders and other joint pains are common ways in which our unconscious draws our attention to these buried hurts. It is very common for people to have major emotional releases of buried pains when receiving spiritual healing or bioenergy interventions for these joint pains, with complete resolution of the pains. With WHEE the emotional releases are as deep and as thorough, but the intensity of the experienced releases is much gentler.

Psychological problems may likewise contribute to causing or worsening headaches, backaches, irritable bowel syndrome, asthma, and other pains and allergic problems. The release of the associated emotional pains will often alleviate and may even cure these physical pains and problems.

Treatment of PTSD with WHEE provides rapid, deep, and lasting relief of symptoms. What is appreciated is that a person can use WHEE whenever symptoms arise. Complete recovery from PTSD may occur fairly rapidly when the original trauma was a single incident, such as an accident or a single episode of abuse, particularly if the trauma was recent. Technically, this is labeled "simple trauma." With long-standing or "complex trauma," in which the abuse was repeated over extended periods, treatment may take months or years, with WHEE addressing multiple issues that rise to consciousness as therapy progresses:

- Anxieties, fears, and terrors triggered by activation of memories of the original trauma
- Angers at the abuser
- Angers at parents or other caregivers who did not provide adequate protection to prevent the abuse

- Deep hurt at having been abused, particularly if the abuser was a family member

- Feelings of guilt over the abused person's imagined responsibility for having invited the abuse

- Feelings of guilt and shame over having felt sexual excitement or other feelings that were aroused in the course of the abuse

- Feelings of betrayal and distrust if the abuser was a parent, trusted relative, caregiver, teacher, priest, or other person who had been trusted

- Feelings of betrayal, frustration, anger, and hurt when caregivers refused to believe the reports of abuse

- Questioning of one's own memory when caregivers refused to believe the reports of abuse

- Shame over revealing sexual abuse or other issues of vulnerability

- Wishes to confront the abuser, for acknowledgment of their wrong-doing and apologies, at the least

- Wanting legal action where it is deemed appropriate for restitution and when the abuser may still be in a position to abuse others

- Being traumatized further by the insensitivities of the legal system

While these steps are outlined in a logical sequence, the unfolding of feelings and retrieval of buried memories has a life and sequence of its own. The course of therapy will vary with each individual, addressing their unique combinations of original traumas, subsequent problems, resistances, personality, relationships, and life circumstances.

Depression

Depression is one of the most insidious and chronic conditions causing psychological pain, and will frequently contribute to or cause physical pains. There are two broad types of depression—hereditary and reactive—which often overlap.

When hereditary depression is present, other members of the family have usually been seriously depressed, suicidal, and/or habitual users of alcohol or street drugs (having self-medicated their pains with these substances). These depressions may be steady and present for long periods of time or may be cyclical, with a waxing and waning that can have intervals varying from hours (not very common) to days, weeks, months, and years. There is often a lack of energy, tiredness, loss of appetite, and difficulty feeling emotions other than depression.

Some hereditary depressions alternate with periods of wildly high moods called mania, during which people are grandiose, hyperactive, need very little sleep, have racing thoughts, and believe they can manage far more than they actually are able to. During these periods they also tend to have very poor judgment and may make foolish decisions, such as poor investments or irresponsible commitments to new relationships. This is called a bipolar (manic-depressive) disorder. Some people with hereditary bipolar disorders only have cyclical depressions, without periods of mania.

Reactive depressions occur in response to difficult situations, such as a death or other loss of relationship with someone close, or the loss of a job, possessions, capacity to function in life (as with injuries and pains that leave a person disabled), or hoped-for prospects. Buried angers at others or at oneself may fester in the unconscious mind, producing reactive depression.

Both kinds of depression often lead to vicious circles of depressed feelings → lessened activities → lessened positive experiences and lessened joy in life → hopelessness → more depressed feelings. The worst-case scenario is a suicide.

I digress here to add a few words on this very serious topic. If as a therapist or as a family member, friend, or colleague you suspect that someone is pondering the possibility of ending their life, it is very important to find a way to open this topic for discussion. People unfamiliar with serious depression may fear that talking about it might encourage a person to act on their suicidal ideas. The opposite is the case. People who can talk with someone about it are less likely to kill themselves. This degree of depression may be handled best by a professional counselor or psychotherapist. Telephone help lines are available 24–7, and it is wise to be sure a person who is seriously depressed knows one of these numbers.[8]

Ted was naturally upset when he lost his middle-management job in electronics due to downsizing after a merger. He

___
[8] For further discussion about suicide, see Chapter 6.

had worked in the same company for over 20 years and had excellent job ratings and references, yet he became depressed when he reached his eightieth resume rejection over a period of six months. It became harder and harder for him to get up in the morning and continue his search for another job.

At home, he was increasingly irritable, crabby, and withdrawn. His wife, too, was beginning to be irritable with him and for the first time in their marriage they had a serious argument that came close to leading them to separate.

Yet it wasn't until Ted found himself starting to self-medicate with increasing numbers of alcoholic drinks every evening that he caught himself in this downward spiral and sought counseling.

Both hereditary and reactive depressions my lead people to self-medicate with alcohol or street drugs and food. These often produce temporary relief through sedation or a brief elevation of mood, but almost always are followed by worsening of depression. Knowing or having available no other remedies, people may become trapped in a second vicious circle of depression → using habituating and addicting substances → more depression → more self-medication.

I drank to drown my pain, but the damned pain learned how to swim, and now I am overwhelmed by this decent and good behavior.

—Frida Kahlo

People with bipolar disorders and moderate or serious reactive depressions that last a long time may do poorly if they do not have anti-depressant medications. While one must always beware of the risks of unwanted effects from medications, there are times when one may find that the best odds are in favor of the medications. Many people also respond to nutritional changes, vitamins and supplements, and/or light therapy (for seasonal depression), which usually require a caregiver with special expertise in this area (a rare commodity).

Changes in hormones and metabolism can also produce depression. Women can often testify to this vulnerability in the days prior to their menses and during menopause. Low thyroid hormone and diabetes may be associated with depression. The rebalancing of the relevant metabolic factors will often clear these depressions.

WHEE can be enormously helpful to people with depression—for addressing limiting beliefs, negative self-image and other pieces of vicious circles, cravings (if they have been comfort eating or self-medicating with street drugs or alcohol), and particularly for memories of traumas that precipitated reactive depression.

The psychological pains of depression are often found to be linked with physical pains. I have many times seen headaches and backaches that revealed underlying depressions as we worked on the physical pains. In some cases these were ways that the unconscious mind was asking for more caring, touch, and other ways of addressing closeness deficits in unsatisfactory relationships. In some people the pains were manifestations of anger at the partner or family member who was not satisfying their needs; in others the pain manifested out of anger at themselves for acts of commission or omission, disappointments, or feelings of guilt or inadequacy. When the psychological dynamics become clear, WHEE often offers rapid relief of these pains.

More often than not, depression has roots in earlier years as well as in the reasons identified in present circumstances. Unresolved grief is a very common factor, along with a history of depression in the adults with whom people lived when they were children. Depression may predispose people to develop pains due to stresses that are not discharged in healthy ways. Bundling these earlier issues with the current ones provides deeper relief of psychological pains and any associated physical ones.

Inflicting Pain

Inflicting pain is often a part of post-traumatic stress disorders. People with PTSDs are easily agitated and angered and often have temper problems. People who have been abused sexually have a much higher likelihood of sexually abusing others.

> Of all the animals, man is the only one that is cruel. He is the only one that inflicts pain for the pleasure of doing it.

> —Mark Twain

This re-enactment occurs because people who are unconscious of the roots of their PTSDs have an inner drive to release their buried hurts, but at the same time are terrified of doing so because their meta-programs block their awareness. These blocks were put in place at the time of the traumas, when the pains and fears were experienced as overwhelming. At that time, burying the feelings and memories was a good choice, preventing further suffering. In later years, however, the blocking beliefs prevent the awareness and release of the hurts. Under these circumstances, some of the buried pains and fears find release through changing the victim into a perpetrator.

Being in a close relationship with another person can become a trigger to this process of releasing buried PTSDs. The very fact that another person is showing that they care for the PTSD sufferer may trigger memories of not having had anyone who cared, which then brings out the old hurts, displaced angers from early years of deprivations or abuse, and fears of losing the present-day caring.

When people with PTSDs want to establish healthier patterns of behavior and relationships, WHEE can be enormously helpful.[9]

Getting Support for Dealing with Pain

Whether joy or sorrowful, the heart needs a double, because a joy shared is doubled and a pain that is shared is divided.

—Ruckett

While each of us, ultimately, has to deal with our own pains, it is enormously helpful to have the help of others to cope. We may be mired in a rut of habits—ways of perceiving, experiencing, and responding to our pains—so that we do not conceive of better ways to deal with them. We may be worn down with the stress and agonies of pains and weary with seeking help to deal with them. We may have anxieties, fears, hurts, angers, depression, and other feelings that leave us feeling drained or overwhelmed. The presence and reflections of a trusted relative, friend, or counselor can be enormously helpful.

The mere presence of a caring person can be one of the best possible remedies. As a caring person, be aware that the healings you bring may be received best as gifts that you offer, not prescriptions that you dictate. Your ways of understanding and dealing with pain may be wonderful new insights to the person who is stuck in suffering; they may, however, be perceived as a lack of understanding of the pain or as your

---

[9] More on this, including clinical examples, in Chapter 3.

being critical of how the other person is dealing with the pain. This is a delicate issue and may sometimes be handled best by a professional therapist who is familiar with pain management.

Conventional medicine is not to be overlooked in treatment of diseases and pain management. When pain medications are well tolerated, they are a blessing. Optimal choices in medications and dosing are essential. A specialist in pain medications may be able to help when problems arise. WHEE can be helpful in reducing side effects of medications, with such affirmations as:

- "Even though I have [nausea/headaches/other side effects] from my medication(s), I still love..."
- "I take my medications and enjoy their benefits, and I love..."[10]

Asking for help and support is important. You may have particular needs that you are unable to meet because of your pain. Asking may be difficult if you have chronic pain, as you may hesitate to become a burden on family and friends. This is a natural situation for using WHEE—converting a worry about this issue (with emotional overlays) into a concern (an appropriate need expressed without emotional attachments).

Accepting help and support is important. It may be a challenging adjustment to realize and accept that you cannot do everything you used to do, before your pains and the problems causing the pains became intense. Often, a significant aspect of pain is that it reminds us to take it easy with some part of our body that is injured or ailing. Listening to and respecting what our body is telling us is an important component of WHEE.

Rejecting offers of advice and help that do not feel helpful may be important as well. There are well-meaning people who may not understand pain in general or your pains in particular. They may suggest that you are not doing enough to deal with your problems, that you are to blame for having your pains, or that your suffering must be a punishment from God for your sins.

How much you heed such observations will depend on your trust in those who are offering such advice. We have seen in earlier parts

---

[10] More on such affirmations in the following chapter.

of this chapter that it is possible to contribute to developing our pains and to relieving them through how we manage stress. There may be a measure of truth in some of these observations. They may, however, contain a measure of misunderstanding about pain in general and about your pains in particular. You must use your good judgment and intuition as to how much to accept such observations and how much to ignore them.

My personal belief is that God never punishes us with pains. We do this to ourselves if we have reasons to feel anxious or guilty about acts or omissions where we feel we might have done better. We can take responsibility for exploring, understanding, and dealing with our problems. We need not feel blamed when suggestions are made—with good intent to help us—that we might consider the ways in which we are stressing ourselves and thereby increasing our pains.

Again, WHEE can be helpful in releasing whatever excess of worry we feel about such issues, allowing us to address them as appropriate concerns.

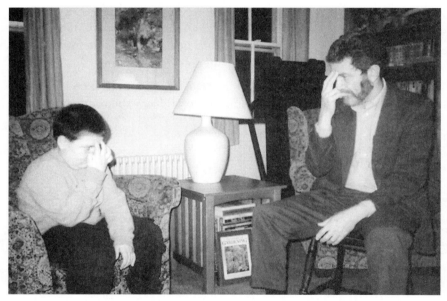

Dr. Benor teaching WHEE using the eyebrow points.

3

The WHEE Method

Pain is a choice, and suffering is optional.

—Anonymous

In the introduction I presented a basic, general description of WHEE. These are the generic details. You may wish to review those basics now, as an orientation to the more detailed discussion that follows.

WHEE is designed to be as flexible as possible in order to fit the preferences and needs of every WHEE user and practitioner. Everything in this book is meant to be a suggestion, not a rule. Although these suggestions are based on forty-five years of practicing psychotherapy and seven years of exploring the ways that WHEE works best, they are most relevant to my own ways of working. I encourage you to adapt WHEE to your own styles of working, and, if you are a therapist, to invite clients to be flexible in their explorations and discover their own best ways for using WHEE.

Broken down to its most basic components, the WHEE method consists of describing the qualities of a pain, assessing its intensity, identifying psychological issues that are associated with the origins and worsening of the pain, tapping alternately on points on the right and left sides of the body while "reprogramming" the body/mind with affirmations and replacement statements, reassessing, and, if necessary, repeating this series of steps until the intensity score is zero. The modality itself can be remarkably effective and is very easy to learn. However, it is important to gain a deeper understanding of the method and its mechanisms—as well as the root causes of the presenting pain—in order to achieve optimal results.

Taking a Thorough Look at One's Life History

The great thing about this world is not so much where we are, but in what direction we are moving.

—Oliver Wendell Holmes, Jr.

If you are a therapist, you are probably eager to get into the technicalities of using WHEE. However, the thorough exploration of your client's history cannot be emphasized enough as the most important first step in the WHEE method. This will very often provide essential clues and suggestions for ways in which WHEE can be used for maximal benefit.

The issues and life problems that can lead to pain are often far more complex than they might appear on the surface. Pains are often the body's way of alerting people to overlooked, stressful psychological challenges in their lives, and are usually related to unconscious feelings and beliefs or disbeliefs. Because we are all unique individuals with our own specific experiences and tendencies, these issues manifest in many ways and as many different kinds of pain. One person may be plagued or even crippled by pains due to physical causes; another may be anxious about the losses of function associated with their pains; a third may be painfully shy and unable to form intimate partnerships; while a fourth may have limiting beliefs that block actualization of their full inner potentials—creating tensions that manifest as, or contribute to, the worsening of pains.

The reasons for the sensitivity around each of these issues will almost always be found in the personal history. A careful, neutral listener may be able to identify those issues from the past that are relevant to the presenting problems much more readily than the people with the problems may be able to do for themselves. This will be illustrated in the following examples and case histories of using WHEE with the help of a therapist.

Safety Issues

Only a fool tests the depth of the water with both feet.

—African Proverb

Safety comes first. I strongly advise you to do only that which feels right and proper for you to do. Do not do anything that is suggested in this book, nor in any other setting, nor by any other authority if it does not feel right to you. There is no single way of helping or healing that works for everyone. If one method does not work for you, there will be others that will help.

Invite your unconscious mind and higher self to protect you when you start any journey of exploration. A simple affirmation or prayer can focus your mind and set the intent for safe healing. Here are several examples of affirmations for self-protection:

- "I accept only that which is for my highest good."
- "I ask [God/Christ/Mary/Buddha/Allah/my higher self/my guardian angels] to protect me as I do this work."
- "May [God/the Infinite Source/All that Is], who made me, make me well, as I am meant to be."

Respect your own inner defenses. You developed these during times of stress, when they protected you from your anxieties, fears, pains, and distress. Out of habit, your unconscious mind believes that these defenses are still necessary. It is helpful to connect with your pains or other issues and dialogue with them, to be certain that your inner self is ready to release them. Ways to do this are discussed in detail, later in this book.

Ground Yourself Regularly

Right-brain intuition that's unanchored in the words of the left hemisphere is like someone who wants to be the conductor of a symphony without knowing how to read or write music. Intuition without grounding in the world is helpful to no one.

—Mona Lisa Schulz

When we explore transpersonal/spiritual dimensions we can easily lose touch with physical reality. You may know people who are grounded as being flighty, erratic in their everyday activities and relationships, or sometimes described as "airy fairy." Grounding ourselves by connecting with the earth and with our physical selves enables us to maintain a healthy balance between the physical and energetic/spiritual worlds, and helps to keep us from getting lost in these other dimensions —allowing us to draw nurturance from these dimensions in order to make our lives on the physical plane more balanced and whole. Breathing and bioenergetic exercises, Yoga, t'ai chi, qigong, jogging, and imagery meditations of linking with Gaia are some of the many ways to ground ourselves. Regular use of some of these practices is strongly recommended. In addition, if we feel we are becoming ungrounded, spacey, or unsure of our centeredness, pausing to use some of these exercises can put us back on track.

The simplest of exercises for grounding connect us to our bodies through our breathing. The metronome of the breath is always with us, and can serve as a focus for concentration.

Exercise: Sit in a quiet place where you will not be interrupted. Watch your breath coming in and going out. Any time a thought, emotion, or physical sensation crosses your awareness, gently let it go and return to focusing on your breathing. With practice, this will help you be present in the moment, fully connected and centered in your body, emotions and mind.

Wholistic healing invites us to open to every level of our being. Our breath can be a pathway to these connections, once we are thoroughly grounded. Breathing awareness can be expanded in various directions to bring you into harmony with your spirit as well as with your body, mind, and emotions.

Exercise: Each molecule and atom of the air we breathe has been present on our planet for billions of years. It has been circulated through all living persons, animals, plants, and other organisms on our planet. We breathe in molecules that were in the breath of Christ, Buddha, Mohammed, and every other being on our planet. As you breathe, focus your awareness on being one with all that lives on our planet.

> **Exercise:** Become aware that, along with oxygen, your breath brings in cosmic energy to nurture and heal every aspect of your being. Connect with your biological energy field, which surrounds and interpenetrates your body, allowing your breath to bring energies to your biofields as well.

> **Exercise:** Use your breath to connect with the Infinite Source, inviting your higher self/spirit/soul to sense your connection with the All.

The knowledge that we are one with a larger whole can help us to put a healing frame around our pains.

Focusing Clearly on the Problem

If we do not know what port we're steering for, no wind is favorable.

—Seneca

The *setup* or *focusing statement* used at the beginning of a round of WHEE is extremely important. This statement must include all the relevant psychological and physical feelings, along with their associated thoughts and memories. Take your time in formulating the best, most precise statement possible. Always remember that the unconscious mind is extremely literal. It will respond willingly to your uses of WHEE, but will be listening to the exact words you use and responding to these words alone. If you do not state exactly what you mean, you cannot assume that, just because it is your own unconscious mind, it will know how you really intend it to focus on your issue.

> Bill was working on his fear of speaking in public. His SUDS was not changing with the statement, "Even though I'm afraid of speaking in public..." After giving this a think, he shifted to, "Even though I'm afraid of how people will respond to what I say..." and the SUDS immediately started going down.

Bill's unconscious knew it wasn't the speaking he was afraid of. Bill was quite an eloquent speaker, with a lot of success in his work as a teacher and in his second career as standup comedian. His successes, however, had been marred by severe anxiety that he had to fight very hard to overcome. His problem was the anxieties he felt about being criticized and rejected.

This is one of the most important parts of the WHEE process. The challenge is to identify the key issue, or collection of issues, of the problem you wish to address. The more you are directly on target, the more effective the whole process will be. Don't worry, though, if you are only partly on target when you start. As you go through the steps of WHEE, you will have the internal feedback you need in order to sharpen your focus.

It is important to write down the precise words you use to describe your issue. If you are on target, you will find the negativity decreasing and you may want to repeat the process until it is all gone. If a certain way of stating your issue has worked, it is very helpful to repeat the exact same words so that it continues to decrease. If you are somewhat off target, the intensity may not diminish. In that case, it is helpful to have your exact words so that you can tweak the way you describe and connect with the problem focus, thereby making WHEE more effective.

Here are some examples of being off-target and sharpening of the problem focus:

- "I feel angry at my son for never cleaning his room."

Sharper focus: "I'm ready to tear my hair out from having to shout and scream at my son to get him to clean his room, when he knows I'm in pain from my migraines and I can't always get on his case the way I should, and his father just sits back and does nothing, leaving it all to me."

- "I'm embarrassed to ask my doctor for different pain pills again."

Sharper focus: "I cringe when I think of complaining that these pain pills aren't working either, after having problems with two other pills as well. My doctor will think I'm a pain in the ass and won't want to see me any more."

- "My backache is worrying me because it's getting worse."

Sharper focus: "I'm terrified because my doctor scheduled an MRI scan since the pain is worsening, and he said he just wanted to be sure it isn't a growth of some sort causing it, and I really, really, really hope this isn't cancer."

The more graphic you can be in describing the issues, the better WHEE can help you decrease their intensity and negativity. As you go through rounds of WHEE, you may connect more graphically and intensely with new words and issues that are related to your original statement of the problem focus. Add these to your original statement and continue using WHEE on the whole list.

As the intensity of your problem focus gets lower with rounds of WHEE, some of the issues on the list may no longer feel relevant. It is fine to drop these and just focus on the remaining, juicy ones.

The SUDS and SUSS

We are healed of a suffering only by expressing it to the full.

—Marcel Proust

Prior to each round of WHEE—whether working directly on an issue or installing a replacement positive—you will find it helpful to check how strongly you believe and feel the negative or replacement positive statement.

I recommend using the *Subjective Units of Distress Scale* (SUDS), in which you rate the intensity of your negative focus on a scale from zero (not bothering you at all) to 10 (the worst it could possibly feel).

After tapping for a few minutes, check the SUDS again. It will usually go down. Repeat the assessing and tapping until it is zero. Anything at all that is higher than a zero is a hedge against truly and completely letting go of an issue. I strongly recommend doing a thorough search for sharper phrasing of the focus, searching for related issues, meta-issues, core beliefs, or other resistances that are blocking your complete release of the problem.

Usually, we aim for an end point of zero on the SUDS scale. If our negative focus is even a fraction of a unit above zero, this often signifies that we are not fully ready to release the issue. Further explorations and work with WHEE on the reasons for not releasing the issue completely are recommended.

Once the SUDS level is down all the way to zero, I recommend installing a *replacement positive statement* to replace the negative that has been released. Prior to installing the replacement positive, and after each round of WHEE to strengthen it, you will find it helpful to check how strongly you believe and feel the replacement positive statement to be true, where zero is "not at all" and 10 is "it couldn't be stronger or firmer." This is the *Subjective Units of Success Scale* (SUSS).

As with everything in WHEE, there are exceptions to all recommendations and no rules written in stone. There are several situations in which installing a replacement positive may be helpful before the SUDS is down to zero.

- With severe PTSD, it may be helpful to park the issue being addressed and install a replacement positive when strong resistance is encountered.

- With serious, chronic depression it may be very helpful to install positives as one of the first uses of WHEE. This helps people to overcome their inertia and lack of motivation to work on their depression.

- When people are frustrated with their difficulties in overcoming cravings or obsessive ruminations on negative self-talk, parking the issue being addressed and installing positives can encourage hope and persistence in continuing to work on the challenging issues.

When people are in a more positive space after installing positives, it will usually be possible to return to the parked issues and proceed to bring the SUDS down to zero.

The SUDS and SUSS provide measures of the intensity of feelings and issues that you are working on. They allow you to sense how quickly you are shifting to release the negatives and to install the positives. They alert you when some part of you is resisting change, so that you can figure out ways to release or get around the resistances.

Some people find their SUDS and SUSS shifting slowly and gradually, perhaps half a number or one number at a time. Others find that their numbers shift in jumps, such as starting at a SUDS of 8 and dropping in one round to 4 or even to 1 or zero. Even for the same person, this usually varies to some degree from one issue to another, and from one phrasing of the focus to another. Our unconscious releases at its own pace, so be patient and just take your rates of shift as indications of the intensity of feelings and of the ability, readiness, or reluctance of your unconscious to release the specific negatives and absorb the positives you have chosen to work on.

At times, the intensity of the SUDS may increase—particularly as you first begin to work on an issue. This is a positive sign. It indicates that you are connecting more strongly with the issue, and that your unconscious mind is allowing more of the negative feelings to surface to consciousness. As you continue to tap, the SUDS numbers will go down.

A *round* of WHEE involves tapping on an issue after checking the SUDS or SUSS, then checking the SUDS or SUSS again to see how much the negative has been released, or how much the replacement positive has been strengthened. A *series* of WHEE includes as many rounds as are needed from the initial negative point to the final positive point.

Children release their pain and other issues much more quickly than adults do, because they haven't had the time to grow barnacles of resistances on their problems like adults have. However, children in pain or distress may not be old enough to assess their inner states, or might not know their numbers yet. They can still measure their SUDS and SUSS by answering the question, "How big is your pain/upset?" by showing a small, medium, or large space between their hands.

The SUDS and SUSS can also be helpful to people who are unused to connecting with and identifying their feelings. With just a little patience and persistence, learning to asses the levels of intensity of their SUDS and SUSS helps them make these connections. Using muscles testing is a further help as it connects them with their feelings and because the practice of assessing feelings helps people to connect with intuition and inner guidance. Muscle testing will be explained toward the end of this chapter.

Physical Sensations as Another Measure of Intensity

Our own physical body possesses a wisdom which we who inhabit the body lack.

—Henry Miller

When we focus on an issue, we often (but not always) experience tensions, aches, pains, or other sensations in various parts of the body. If physical pain itself is the focus, then the pain may actually increase as you focus, especially early in the series of tapping. It is helpful to do

SUDS assessment on these sensations, either individually or collectively, if there are more than one.

These sensations also serve as markers for the intensity of your issue and for your progress in releasing the negatives. Usually, the physical sensations will dissipate more quickly than your feelings about the issue. If the physical sensations persist when your issues SUDS for the emotional components reaches zero, it is best to continue using WHEE until the SUDS for the sensations reaches zero as well. If you find that your physical sensations resist releasing, you can deal with them using the approaches described below for resistances, or you may choose to dialogue with the sensations to discover what your unconscious wants to tell you.

Tapping

If you can learn from hard knocks, you can also learn from soft touches.

— Carolyn Gilmore

Alternating right and left stimulation of the body, in and of itself, will bring about releases of anxieties, stress, pain, negative beliefs, and whatever else you would like to let go of. This has been amply demonstrated in clinical EMDR experience and confirmed in EMDR research.

Any alternating right and left stimulation of the body may be used:

- You may tap the ends of your eyebrows, nearest the bridge of your nose. These points are convenient for tapping with the index finger and middle finger of one hand, or can be tapped with the index finger of right and left hands. These eyebrow points are extra-helpful as they are also acupressure releasing points (used in EFT).

- You may cross your arms and pat each arm with the opposite hand. This is called the *butterfly hug*.

- You may pat your thighs with your hands, or tap them with a finger of each hand as you hold your hands on your lap.

- You may alternate tapping your feet on the floor.

- You may alternate tightening the toes of your right foot and then your left foot. Some people find this a more potent method if they do it standing up.

- You may alternate tapping your teeth with your tongue, right and left, right and left.

The last four tapping methods offer varying degrees of privacy, which can be beneficial should you be in situations where you would rather not be noticed doing WHEE. In these cases, you would recite the affirmations silently to yourself.

A particularly potent method for tapping is to alternate right and left tapping with your feet while at the same time tapping with your hands on your right and left sides — but on the opposite side to the side you are tapping with your feet. This is similar to a method called *cross crawling* used in a method called Brain Gym for harmonizing right and left brain hemispheres, described by Dennison and Dennison.

EMDR started with alternating eye movements to right and left. While this works well, some people suffer from dizziness, vertigo, or nausea if they do it for any length of time. EMDR has also developed stereo cassette tapes with alternating right and left ear stimulation, but this tethers a user to a cassette player and therefore reduces the flexibility of its use.

Affirmations

To understand the heart and mind of a person look not at what he has already achieved but at what he aspires to.

—Kahil Gibran

Any positive cognition (thought, belief, image, feeling memory, or so forth) can be used to counteract and neutralize the negativity of an unpleasant cognition. I have found that about nine out of ten people are comfortable with "I love and accept myself, wholly and completely." If this statement doesn't feel right or fit with their belief system, however, I always tell people to replace it with one that does. Here are some other counteracting affirmations that people have preferred, and which have proven to be good for working with children:

- "I love myself a lot."
- "I remember my mother cuddling me with love when I was [little/younger]."
- "I know that my family loves and accepts me."
- "I remember the [time/feelings] of [a positive experience]."
- "I feel safe now." (This is especially useful for children removed from abusive settings.)

The body participates in holding memories and in releasing them, as witnessed by rapid reductions in pains through the use of dialogue. We can use the mind-emotions-body connections within the WHEE process—and thereby enhance its efficacy—by adding the following to any affirmation:

- "I hereby release all of this pain/distress/trauma/memory from every cell and particle and fiber of my being, and I love and accept myself…"

WHEE can also relieve insomnia, which often accompanies serious pains. Clients have reported rapid, complete cures of their inability to fall asleep upon going to bed and if they wake up during the night. This is one instance where a SUSS is unnecessary, for obvious reasons. However, if people are anxious about not being able to fall asleep then they can work on the anxiety itself, in which case a SUSS is helpful.

Another way to release pain and other physical and psychological problems, and at the same time connect more strongly with spiritual aspects of ourselves, is by shifting our habits of perceiving ourselves as separate from the greater world around us. Here is a further affirmation that can help with this process of expanding awareness, while facilitating releases of pains and other issues:

- "I hereby release any and all traces of this issue from every energetic portion and aspect of my being…"

Within the wholistic framework we come to appreciate that we have a bioenergetic body as well as a physical body; that we are related to other people and other aspects of the world through collective consciousness; and that spiritual aspects of ourselves connect us with spiritual dimensions of reality outside ourselves. These ways of understanding our relationships with the world around us can significantly potentiate our uses of WHEE.

Counteracting spiritual affirmations can also provide a palpably stronger boost to the affirmation process. To any of the above you might add:

- "...and [God/Christ/Mary/Buddha/Allah/the Infinite Source/the Divine] loves and accepts me, wholly and completely and unconditionally."

- "I experience myself as one with [all of Nature/the cosmos]..."

Just as buried feelings and memories from our present life can cause pains and other problems in our wellbeing, so can unresolved issues from past lives, which comprise another facet of our spiritual selves. A generic affirmation to release these could be:

- "I hereby release any and all traces of this issue that arises from any and all past life residues, and I love..."

Yet another part of our spiritual selves can include memories of traumatic experiences from parents, grandparents, and other family members with which we connect unconsciously. We might acquire these through family myths or habits of beliefs and practices, or through energetic patterns in which our family collectively participates. A generic affirmation to release these could be:

- "I hereby release any and all negative memories and residues contributing to my pains that might be found in my genetic inheritance, cellular memories, biological energy fields, family memories, and karma, and I love..."

Explanations and illustrations for how such wholistic applications can be used as parts of the WHEE process can be found in later chapters of this book, in case any of these are unclear or seem far-fetched.

Many other Energy Psychology systems commonly suggest shortcuts in using affirmations, such as tapping on one point or through a series of points while saying, "All of this problem," and relying on the tapping to release the negative problem focus. WHEE specifically recommends using the full affirmation each time rather than any abbreviation. By continuing to repeat the full problem focus we invite the process to unfold with further sharpening of our statements.

The full affirmation is especially helpful where a spiritual component is included, as it invokes spiritual energies to enhance the effects of the affirmation. At the same time, it strengthens our connection with our spiritual awareness. For this reason as well, affirmation shortcuts are not recommended.[1]

Replacement Positive Statement

> *If you don't like something, change it. If you can't change it, change your attitude.*
>
> —Maya Angelou

Once the SUDS level is down to zero, it is helpful to install a *replacement positive statement* to take the place of the negative that has been released. When a replacement positive is in place, it is much harder for the negative to return.

For instance, if you have released a negative memory of being in an accident (which can contribute to the persistence of pains following the event), you might start tapping and say something like: "I can recall the accident and feel comfortable with the memory." Then you add, "and I love and accept myself, wholly and completely."

Here are other examples of replacement positive statements:

- "I look back on the [experience of my pain/unsuccessful treatments of my pain/fears of recurring pain] and feel comfortable with my progress…"

- "I recall my [mother/father/other significant person] having pain and feel at peace with the memory and myself today…"

- "I forgive myself for my [lack of self-care/lack of persistence/procrastination] in dealing with my pain…"

The replacement positive statement is very personal and must be individualized to match your situation and feelings about it. You may need to take some time to explore a variety of positives before you find one that feels like a good match for your situation, beliefs, and feelings. I have seen several people take a week or more to sort out their replacement positives, particularly after releasing feelings from severe PTSDs. Here are some examples of these affirmations:

- "I know my father was abused by his father when he was little, and he never had anyone to help him deal with his feelings from his PTSD…"

---

[1] For more on the spiritual aspects of WHEE, see Chapters 6 and 7.

- "While I would never have chosen to be raped in order to learn these lessons, I have become a much more deeply aware and compassionate person through my therapy to deal with my feelings from the rape..."

- "Because I [had that nasty accident/got cancer/suffered these terrible pains], I met some wonderful people who have helped me transform my life — way beyond dealing with my [injuries/illness/pains]..."

It is absolutely essential to phrase the replacement positive statement in positive terms. The unconscious mind does not absorb the word "not," so a statement such as, "I look back on my experience of pain and do not feel upset" is a setup for failure. Your unconscious mind would be hearing, "I look back on my experience of pain and feel upset." In effect, you would be reinstalling a pain reaction to the memory.

Precision in making the replacement positive statements is also important. There is a significant difference between "I *can* look back at..." or "I *can* forgive..." and "I look back at..." or "I forgive...." The second options are full commitments to the positive, while the insertion of "can" may be a hedge that your unconscious accepts as some measure of unreadiness on your part to make the shift and really change, fully letting go of old patterns and accepting/installing new ones.

Writing down the exact words you use is an enormous help in using WHEE. This enables you to trouble-shoot when your SUDS or SUSS are not budging. (More on this below, under *Journaling*.)

The replacement positive is helpful beyond its use to replace a negative that has been released; it is also a way of reprogramming and retraining yourself — of replacing childhood programming, which often focused largely on fighting or fleeing and burying your negative experiences. Have you ever asked yourself, "What is the opposite of a vicious circle?" I find it odd that the English language does not have a commonly used concept for this. (French, German, and Swedish have such terms.) Thus, it is even difficult to think of working in this direction.

The term I use to invite you to work at installing positives in your feelings, beliefs, and habits is *sweetening spiral*. For instance: you may address your stress responses with WHEE → feel less [stress/pain/meta-anxieties about the stress] → experience greater self-confidence in dealing with stress → feel fewer anxieties when confronting the next stress → attain greater confidence yet → and so forth. Figure 2 illustrates a sweetening spiral in using WHEE for pain.

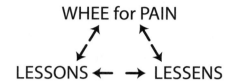

Figure 2. A sweetening spiral with WHEE.

As you practice this, you will find yourself more competent and confident in doing it. You will then have greater success inviting and installing positives into your life because of your experience, successes, and confidence. The concept of the sweetening spiral is like a road map to finding more affirming ways of dealing with yourself and others.

> *No Pessimist ever discovered the secrets of the stars,*
>
> *or sailed to an uncharted land,*
>
> *or opened a new heaven to the human spirit*

> —Helen Keller

You may find it difficult to believe me when I say that it is possible to reach a point where you will welcome upsetting experiences in your life. Yet my experience, both personally and with many people I have helped, is that if you practice WHEE sufficiently, you may come to view difficult experiences as opportunities to clear more of the old hurts, fears, and angers buried in the file drawers and closets and caves of your unconscious mind. Rather than finding such experiences to be negative, daunting, depressing, discouraging, or disappointing, you may find them challenging, exciting, and gratifying. Perhaps this is what the French writer Anaïs Nin was referring to when she wrote that "the secret to joy is the mastery of pain."

Rate, Duration, and Intensity of Tapping

> *Things turn out best for people who make the best out of the way things turn out.*

> —John Wooden

For absolute clarity, let me specify precisely how I recommend the tapping be done: Alternate with one tap on one side of the body, followed by one tap on the opposite side; repeat—back and forth, back and forth.

As with other aspects of WHEE, you are free to adapt your rate and duration of tapping to whatever feels and works best to shift your SUDS and SUSS rates. I have seen people do equally well with tapping as fast as they can or as slowly as one tap in about ten seconds.

Duration is similarly variable. Most people find that tapping a few seconds after the statement of an affirmation and a deep breath is sufficient. Others find that tapping for a minute or two longer feels better and is more productive.

How fast and how long you tap may vary within a session, with the issue, or may shift gradually over a period of time to be regularly longer or shorter. Again, allow your intuition and the rate of shifting in your SUDS and SUSS to guide you.

The intensity or firmness you use in tapping is entirely a matter of your personal preference. Some people like to tap vigorously, while others may tap lightly or just gently touch each side of the body.

Incremental Learning to Find Your Best Ways for Using WHEE

In the pursuit of learning, every day something is acquired. In the pursuit of Tao, every day something is dropped.

—Lao Tsu

In order to get a baseline sense of how fast your affirmation is working with whatever method of tapping you have chosen, it is helpful to start off with a few rounds of WHEE on a difficult issue that goes down slowly. Then change only one element at a time and repeat the same process, noting whether this enhances the rate of release of your SUDS, and whether you notice any qualitative differences as you use the WHEE process. Your body, emotions, and mind will give you feedback on how helpful your new element is in dealing with this issue.

This is one of the most helpful aspects of the WHEE process. Because WHEE is so rapid, it is easy to use it for feedback on elements across the wholistic spectrum, exploring for potential aids in releasing whatever you want to release and in installing replacement positives.

Incremental learning will allow you to appreciate the contributions of spiritual elements in WHEE and in your life. For instance, if you start with the basic counteracting affirmation, "I love and accept myself…" and observe your progress, then add "and the Infinite Source loves and accepts me…" you may notice quantitative and qualitative differences in your progress.[2]

Journaling

> *I wonder if I shall burn this sheet of paper like most others I have begun in the same way....How could I write a diary without throwing upon paper my thoughts, all my thoughts—the thoughts of my heart as well as of my head?—and then how could I bear to look on them after they were written? Adam made fig leaves necessary for the mind, as well as for the body....Well! but I will write: I must write—and the oftener wrong I know myself to be, the less wrong I shall be in one thing—the less vain I shall be!*

> —Elizabeth Barrett Browning

It is extremely helpful to keep careful records of the precise words you use with WHEE, in each round of SUDS and SUSS, because:

- If you interrupt your series of rounds for any reason, this allows you to return to where you were and continue.

- When you have been successful and the numbers are shifting without resistances, it is a help to have the beneficial wording should you ever want to revisit this issue or should you encounter a similar one.

- Examining the precise words you have used may give you clues to how to understand and get around any resistance you might run up against in the future.

Putting your words in writing often gives them a sharper focus. You may pick up items or nuances that escaped your notice when you were saying them mentally or out loud. Similarly, reviewing your journal entries after a pause of a day or more may give you a different perspective on them. I have often found for myself that sleeping on an issue that has been intense will open new understandings and new avenues by

---

[2] Spiritual aspects of WHEE are discussed further in Chapters 6 and 7.

which to address the issues. This is true even when the SUDS reached zero and the SUSS was at zero when I stopped working on an issue.

If you are working with a counselor or in co-counseling, your journal provides a way of sharing specifics and obtaining inputs from the other person. I have been repeatedly surprised how the inputs of another person have shed light on my own issues and on those of my clients—providing insights that we would totally have missed on our own. It is very easy to be in a rut of self-perceptions and conceptualizations so that we miss obvious issues that another person can spot, both in clearing our dross and vicious circles, and in installing positives and creating sweetening spirals.

Journaling also provides a diary for your progress. It is helpful to look back at your journal entries from time to time in order to see in which ways you are changing and growing, or in which ways you may be stuck.

How to Deal with Resistances

Success is the ability to go from one failure to another with no loss of enthusiasm.

—Winston Churchill

Gary Craig introduced me to the label *resistance* for those times when the SUDS is not shifting in response to tapping plus affirmations. In WHEE, the same applies for dealing with the SUSS, as you install a positive replacement for whatever negativity you have released. There are varieties of ways to deal with resistances, as detailed below. I find this feature of WHEE to be extremely attractive—after the other benefits of speed and flexibility that WHEE brings to dealing with problems and transforming beliefs and attitudes.

The easiest way to deal with resistances is by *massaging the collarbone releasing spot* (also called the tender spot or the sore spot). When your SUDS or SUSS number is not shifting after two rounds of tapping, you may choose to do the following:

- Locate your releasing spot, which is just below the midpoint of your collarbone (half way along your collarbone, between your breast bone/sternum and your shoulder).

- Using three fingers of one hand, massage the muscles of your chest just below the midpoint of the clavicle.

- You may choose to massage either side, or may find that it works better for you to massage both sides—either one after the other or simultaneously.

- After massaging your releasing spot, return to using WHEE as usual on your issue.

- Most of the time, I find that this shifts the resistance and facilitates further progress in using WHEE.

Many people find that this spot feels queasy, tender, or even sore to the touch as they are working on a resistance. There is no need to recite an affirmation as you massage this point.

I have found that in most cases, this is like a brake release that allows people to move on with little fuss or bother. This is one of the more remarkable aspects of WHEE (and other meridian based therapies).

An alternative method of tapping may prove more potent with a given issue, or even with the same issue over a period of time. Many people find a favorite, such as the butterfly hug, that is particularly helpful to them and tend to stick with that method. I do not know why, in some cases, one's usual method that has been successful with other issues does not work well, while alternative methods work better.

Adjusting the wording of your focusing statement to deal with resistance is the next step, if massaging the releasing point is not effective. This is why it is important to write down the exact wording of your affirmation or reinforcing statement. Tweaking the words you use in your focusing statement may make an enormous difference in your abilities to release the issues you are working on.

The following are examples of successful tweaks:

- *Resistance with:* "Even though I've had this pain in my back for fourteen years…"

    Successful tweak: "Even though my back pain is excruciating when I bend over even a little, and I'm truly weary of being limited in my activities, including my sex life, for the last fourteen years …"

- ***Resistance with:*** "Even though I'm upset with my doctor for botching up the surgery and leaving me with this pain..."

  Successful tweak: "Even though I'm *furious* with my doctor for botching up the surgery and leaving me with this pain, and wish he had to suffer just a fraction of what I've suffered these three and a half years..."

- ***Resistance with:*** "Even though I have unpleasant side effects from my medications..."

  Successful tweak: "Even though I feel nauseous and get headaches with my chemotherapy, and hate the atmosphere of the hospital where I have to go for the chemo..."

Usually, it helps to be very specific in describing your issues. Detailing the feelings and the issues that are involved may take a little thought. Sometimes others who know you and your situation may add suggestions that you might not think of. This is often true in therapy, where the therapist can make suggestions from experiences of helping other people, as well as from an understanding of psychotherapy in general and of you and your history in particular.

Generic, non-specific affirmations can sometimes be helpful. There may be factors of which we are not fully aware, but that we can guess may be preventing our clearing of issues. By including a generic statement in our setup focus we may be able to clear these. For example: *"I hereby release any and all..."*

- "...reasons why I may not be aware of for holding onto my [pains/other symptoms], and I love and accept myself..."

- "...other negative feelings from experiences I had with my abusive older brother, which may be outside my conscious awareness at this time..."

- "...cravings that I have not cleared yet..."

While it may seem contradictory that both being very specific and being generic in affirmations can be helpful, such is the human condition. No one shoe fits all, and WHEE can be adapted in every possible manner to match the needs and preferences of the individual.

When I trained in conventional, psychodynamic, Freudian psychotherapy, resistances were a focus for work that could take months and years. It is a joy to use WHEE, which rapidly dissipates resistances and allows you to deal with issues and move on with your life.

Earlier, similar experiences may be asking for release along with the issue you are working on. When all of the above methods for dealing with resistance have not helped, or when there is an obvious—or even likely—connection between a current issue and a known traumatic event in the past, it may be helpful to work on the current issue at the same time as you work on the past issue. This is called *bundling*.

Here are examples of bundling issues when working with resistances:

- *Resistance with:* "Even though I have this excruciating tension headache…"

  Successful bundling: "Even though I have this excruciating tension headache and remember how my head hurt for weeks and months after the auto accident when I was eight years-old…"

- *Resistance with:* "Even though I become petrified and have stomach cramps whenever my partner and I get into angry exchanges…"

  Successful bundling: "Even though I become petrified and have stomach cramps whenever my partner and I get into angry exchanges, and this reminds me of my parents fighting with each other and getting angry with me all the time, and my guts getting in an uproar every time that happened…"

- *Resistance with:* "Even though I have pains in my stomach every month with my period that sometimes make me miss work…"

  Successful bundling: "Even though I have pains in my stomach every month with my period that sometimes make me miss work, and it's exactly what happened to my mother…"

- *Resistance with:* "Even though I get migraines, particularly when things are not going well with my partner…"

  Successful bundling: "Even though I get migraines, particularly when things are not going well with my partner and I'm getting the silent treatment, and I remember how my parents ignored me most of the time, except that one time I had a head injury…"

Experiences of traumas in the past, both our own and those of others who were close to us, may often leave deep imprints in the unconscious mind. While the memories and feelings of these events may be buried in the unconscious, they may not be buried deeply enough to avoid being stirred into semi-awareness by another, similar traumatic experience in the present.

While these experiences are often unpleasant, they offer opportunities for clearing out old issues that no longer need to be buried. With time and experience, we may even come to seek out such buried issues when we are clearing current issues—even if these issues that were buried many years earlier do not initially present themselves clearly. This may be particularly helpful with broader, more general experiences of rejection or chronic abuse.

An earlier illustrative example is my clearing of earlier memories of being unwanted by my mother, in the process of clearing my heartache over the ending of a current relationship. It is very common to find ourselves peeling layer after layer of an onion of hurts and tears, over long periods of time.

Meta-anxieties

Unconscious meta-anxieties and beliefs may lead you to hold onto issues and feelings, even when you consciously want to release them.[3] Chronic pains are particularly notorious for creating beliefs and disbeliefs that may make it difficult to release them, but other issues may also create resistances.

- *Resistance with the focus:* "Even though I have these pains in my hands that make it impossible to do the simplest things like washing the dishes…"

   Meta-anxiety: "If I let go of these pains, I'll be stuck again with all of the housework, in addition to my part-time job and caring for the kids…"

- *Resistance with the focus:* "Even though I have these horrendous migraines…"

   Meta-anxiety: "If I stop having these headaches, my partner will stop showing me the tender caring I'm getting now, just like it used to be before I had these migraines…"

---

[3] See Chapter 2 under *Vicious Circles.*

- *Resistance with the focus:* "Even though I'm afraid to speak in public..."

  Meta-anxiety: "If I speak up in front of strangers, I'll only [make a fool of myself/be rejected/ridiculed], just like it happened [in my family/school/church]...

- *Resistance with the focus:* "Even though I procrastinate and avoid [saying/doing the things] that will bring me success..."

  Meta-anxiety: "My father said I'd never amount to anything, so there's no point even trying..."

Some of these meta-anxieties are specific to situations and experiences from the past and present, and some are more general and may interfere in many aspects of our life. It may be obvious and easy to identify the meta-anxieties, or it may require a bit of detective work. Often, meta-anxieties are difficult for us to identify by ourselves, because they are so imbedded in our belief systems that we don't ever question them. In fact, we may not even notice them. A therapist may be of enormous help with these. This presumes, of course, that the therapist does not have blind spots similar to our own.

> *Part of every misery is, so to speak, the misery's...reflection: the fact that you don't merely suffer but have to keep on thinking about the fact that you suffer. I not only live each endless day in grief, but live each day thinking about living each day in grief.*
>
> —C. S. Lewis

Once meta-anxieties and meta-beliefs are identified, WHEE can be used to reduce their intensity just like it is used for the primary level issues. It is then possible to install replacement meta-positives to replace the negatives that have been released.

Another resource for helping you to identify meta-anxieties and beliefs is Asha Clinton's manual for what she calls *core beliefs*. That text includes detailed lists of paired negative beliefs and suggested replacement statements, all categorized under headings such as depression, abuse, control, denial, exploitation, and many more. Here are just a few examples:

- I have nothing to live for/I have my own healing and transformation to live for.

- I don't deserve to be healed/I deserve to be healed.
- I must be perfect/It's plenty good enough to be human.
- I am powerless/My power is real but limited.
- I am the least talented/My talents are within normal limits.
- I don't deserve to be respected/I deserve to respect and be respected.

In some cases the term *core beliefs* is used to designate beliefs that we accepted uncritically and installed in our unconscious minds when we were young, at the developmental stage of absorbing what the world is about. For example, abusive—or even simply misinterpreted—experiences may have been absorbed as: "I could never be loved," or "I am [clumsy/dumb/ugly/unable to be understood]."

Again, it bears repeating that it will be helpful to journal precisely what you have said in your setup statements and affirmations. This may be particularly true for identifying meta-issues, some of which can be challenging to recognize. In addition, when you pause to clarify and clear the resistances of your meta-anxieties, your journal entries will bring you right back to where you left off in working on the primary issues. Journaling the meta-issues you address may also prove to be a help in the future, should you encounter similar resistances with other primary issues.

The release of meta-anxieties and beliefs is often experienced as scary business because the unconscious mind may hold meta-meta-beliefs, such as:

- It is not safe to let go of these beliefs that have helped me avoid feeling the buried hurts and fears.
- I will [fall apart/not be able to tolerate/suffer beyond my ability to survive] if I agree to release these buried hurts and fears.

WHEE can be used to release these limiting meta-meta beliefs. While at first it feels scary to do so, it becomes easier and easier with practice. With time, it can actually become a relief to know that you have a method for dealing even with these very scary parts of your unconscious childhood programming. As new issues arise in your life that invite you to use WHEE on them, you may come to look forward to clearing such meta-feelings and meta-beliefs from the past, along with your current issues.

Worry vs. Concern

Converting worries into concerns may be a shortcut to releasing blocking issues or starting a sweetening spiral. In many cases it helps to ask oneself, "Would it be okay to change these anxieties (or meta-anxieties/fears/worries) into concerns?" This is like the difference between addressing issues as the archetypal film worrier, Woody Allen, would do, vs. addressing them like the archetypally calm and logical Mr. Spock from Star Trek does. If clients are not familiar with these examples, I ask whether they could identify with the difference between how Eeyore might respond ("Oh, me! Oh, my! This is terrible!") vs. how Christopher Robin would ("So, Pooh, what shall we do now to fix this?").

This is, in WHEE terms, the installation of a positive meta-belief/attitude to replace a negative one. I have been pleasantly surprised at how easily many people are able to do this.

Imagery and dreams may open doorways into helpful releases of deep issues with the help of WHEE. Working on dream imagery, such as the figure of a monster in a nightmare, can connect with all of the elements of past hurts, anxieties, fears, angers, and other feelings that the unconscious mind combined into the monster figure. We can do the same with any image created from our imagination to represent an issue, problem or relationship in the present or from the past that we wish to address. Often, using WHEE to focus on images in this way can produce profound healings because they carry the healing to all of the elements that relate to the image.

Patience and persistence may be required in dealing with challenging situations, particularly where there is a history of repeated traumas. Peeling the onion of resistances may seem at times to be an endless proposition. With patience and persistence, improvements will occur. The help of a therapist may be required for resolution of some of the more stubborn resistances, but the result will be well worth the effort. As Jim Rohn said, "We must all suffer from one of two pains: the pain of discipline or the pain of regret. The difference is discipline weighs ounces while regret weighs tons."

Bundling and Partializing

The challenge is honoring our uniqueness as we learn how "to listen to ourselves as if we were listening to a message from the universe."

— S. A. Conn

A variety of examples were given above, but this subject deserves a few words of further clarification.

Some issues may respond better when they are bundled. That is, when every element that is relevant to the issue is named as the focus for a WHEE series, the SUDS and SUSS may shift more rapidly and easily. It is sometimes surprising how many different items can be emptied from the same file drawer in a WHEE series!

- *Initial issue:* "Even though I am angry with my boss for overlooking me in the last round of promotions…"

  Additional elements bundled with the initial issue: "…and I'm still mad at him for trashing my last report; and for how he brought Milly, my secretary, to tears over a few typing errors…"

- *Initial issue:* "Even though I am deeply hurt because my husband forgot our anniversary…"

  Additional elements: "…and for not giving our relationship priority [ahead of his career/going out with the boys]; and for leaving me to do most of the chores, even though I have a salaried job, too…"

- *Initial issue:* "Even though I feel guilty for burdening my family with my limitations due to the arthritis…"

  Additional elements: "…and I vowed when I was growing up that I would never burden anyone like my mother did when she was severely depressed, and I ended up being a parentified child, caring for my younger sister and brother…"

Other issues may respond better when the focus is narrower. That is, you might choose to work on a single element at a time within a complex issue. I call this *partializing.*

- *Initial issue:* "Even though my irritable bowel acts up when I eat greasy or very spicy foods, and reacts with cramps when I'm nervous or angry…"

Partialized: Addressing each element separately, possibly bundling some of the psychological issues but using WHEE with the physical irritants separately.

- *Initial issue:* "Even though I have horrible tension headaches when I'm angry with my wife, and I know it started in childhood when I was angry with my mother but didn't dare say anything, and it was worsened when I had the whiplash injury…"

Partialized: Addressing each element separately. Within each separate category, however, there may be other elements that would respond well to WHEE when bundled.

Bundling or partializing can be done at any time in a series, even when several rounds have already been started with a narrower or broader focus. In fact, when you are dealing with a resistance you may find it helpful at times to shift from partializing to bundling or vice versa.

Here is another example that illustrates many of the methods for dealing with resistances. It also points out that what might seem on the surface like a simple issue may turn out to be the tip of an emotional iceberg that requires much more work to clear than would have been anticipated at first.

Iris worked on her worry about her granddaughter, Grace, who was distressed over the separation and divorce of her parents, Iris's daughter and son-in-law. After Iris brought the SUDS down to zero, I had her check whether the SUDS remained zero if she pictured herself speaking with her granddaughter, and she reported that it rose again to a 4. She cleared that to a zero and proceeded to install a statement of confidence in her ability to be helpful in this situation.

At her next visit, Iris reported with disappointment that she had still been distressed when faced with the actual situation of Grace's upsets with her parents' bitter arguing and fussing with each other. Iris questioned whether WHEE was really effective and had even wondered whether it was worth coming back for further sessions.

It was helpful to Iris to consider the difference between worry and concern. She could then see that what she was after was the release of the worry. With further discussion, she realized that it was really hard for her to let go of feeling responsible for Grace's problems because Iris, too, had been through a troublesome divorce that upset her daughter, Grace's mother. After several rounds of WHEE to clear feelings about these and related issues, Iris felt her SUDS was a more solid zero than at the previous session.

It was also helpful to Iris to work on the meta-issues that were triggered by Grace's distress. These included Iris's lack of self-confidence, feelings of having been a failure as a wife and mother, buried angers at her ex-husband, and recent ones at her son-in-law. The angers brought Iris to explore and release her core beliefs that: expressing anger was something that only "bad" people did (residue of her mother's blaming her father for issues that led to Iris's parents' divorce); and that she, herself, was bad for having contributed to or having caused her parents' divorce. (Children often blame themselves for their parents' problems.) After resolving these issues with WHEE, Iris realized she had nearly run away from therapy rather than re-examine these buried core beliefs around anger and guilt.

My experience has been that with patience and persistence, almost any issue can be helped with WHEE.

Parking an Issue

Patience is a bitter plant that produces sweet fruit.

— Charles Swindoll

You may find that you are working well with an issue and in several rounds of WHEE the SUDS has been going down steadily, but suddenly another issue comes to mind that is much stronger than the one you had started on. When this happens, you may choose to park the first issue and proceed with the one that feels stronger or more important to you. It is helpful to write down the particular words you have been using on the first issue so that you can return to work on it later. If it was shifting well, you will then have the words that worked. If it was not shifting then you may well see ways to tweak your wording when you come back to the issue again after a break.

When working on complex issues you may find that there are ups and downs in your progress with various sub-sections of the issues you are clearing and restructuring. I have found this to be particularly likely when dealing with depression, bereavement, and cravings. Dealing with the intensities of feelings and problems may feel like being on a roller-coaster ride. Knowing and anticipating that this may be the way you experience the WHEE process of self-healing is often a help because then you are not as likely to become discouraged when you've been moving along comfortably but suddenly take an unexpected dip or turn that demands your attention.

Muscle Testing for Dealing with Resistances

Intellect must be balanced by intuition and caring, so that information will be used appropriately, for the good of all and for the future generations.

—Kenneth Cohen

Muscle testing is such a potent method that it deserves a section of its own. It allows us to access our unconscious and intuitive wisdom.

For over 100 years it has been known that we can communicate with the unconscious mind through what is called an *ideomotor response*. A hypnotherapist can instruct hypnotized people to let their unconscious mind answer *yes* by raising the index finger of their right hand, and *no* by raising the index finger of their left hand (or through any other body movements).

Through muscle testing, a therapist will assess the strength of people's muscles. For instance, the therapist will have a person hold their arm straight out to the side at shoulder height, asking the person to resist the therapist's pressing down on their wrist – as a baseline measure of strength. Then the therapist tests their strength immediately after stating a true statement out loud, and again after making a false statement. In most cases, the arm will remain strong with the true statement and will go weak with the false statement. After establishing this baseline of responses, the therapist can then check their muscle response following any statement, such as "I am ready to release all of my pain now," or "I want [or need] to hold onto some of my pain now." People are often very surprised at their own muscle responses, which may indicate the opposite of what they consciously think they want.[4]

Warning: Read all notes and cautions below before using muscle testing!

It is possible to test one's own muscles in order to communicate with one's own unconscious mind. Several approaches are in common use:

The Bi-digital O-ring Test (BDORT)

Hold the tips of your left thumb and little finger together, forming an "O" or ring. Hook your right thumb through this ring, just where the left thumb and finger are touching and see how firmly you have to pull in order to break the grip of these fingers. Now, ask yourself, "What does my *yes* feel like?" and repeat the process, noting any change in the strength of your grip. Repeat the process, checking the strength of your grip while you are asking yourself, "What does my *no* feel like?" Many people will find there is a distinct difference in the strength of their grip with a *yes* and a *no*. Most frequently, people find that the *yes* is stronger.

Index Finger Muscle Testing

While sitting, rest your left hand on your leg, near your knee. Raise your index finger. Use your right index finger to press down on your raised left index finger, to check the strength of your left finger. Now, repeat this while you think of a question that can be answered with a *yes* or a *no*. For instance, you might ask, "Is chocolate good for me?" (You may substitute any other food you have cravings for.) See if you notice any change in the strength of your left index finger. Weakness generally indicates a *no*, strength signifies *yes*.

---

[4] Muscle testing was derived originally from Applied Kinesiology, which uses much more detailed methods to identify specific body dysfunctions that are associated with particular acupuncture meridians.

Thumbnail Muscle Testing

Gently rub your first finger back and forth across the nail of your thumb, while asking "What is my *yes*?" and "What is my *no*?" Note any differences in what you feel with your finger. Extend this to practice with other questions. You might say out loud, "Today is ___" (stating the correct day) and explore the feeling of your finger running across your thumbnail. Then say, "Today is ___" (stating the wrong day) and again check your sensation. The *yes* usually feels smoother, but this is a very individual modality, with a wider range of variations than many other muscle testing approaches.

This method is helpful because it is unobtrusive and can be used in almost any situation, including while driving. This is the method I prefer personally.

Your Arm as Your Indicator

Extend your arm out to your side, parallel with the floor. Have a friend test the strength of your arm muscles by pressing down on your wrist to establish your baseline strength to resist her pushing down. (She should press firmly, but not so hard as to "break" your position.) Think silently to yourself of a situation that makes you feel sad. (Don't tell your friend what you are thinking, so there will be no question that your arm is being pressed down either more or less firmly according to her expectations.) Note whether your muscle strength is different when she pushes down a second time, as you are focused on sadness. Then rest your arm a moment and have her press down on your wrist again while you're thinking of something that makes you happy. Note the strength of your arm.

Sadness usually produces weakness; happiness strengthens the muscles. Occasionally an individual will have a habitually reversed response. A woman I worked with once shared her experience: "I grew up in a tough neighborhood. I taught myself to be tough if I was sad and never to cry, because if I cried they made fun of me." Her arm was much stronger when she was sad.

Some people get no responses from muscle testing of any sort. Other signals can be agreed with your unconscious mind.

Imagery Instead of Muscle Testing

Bring up a blank screen in your mind's eye. Ask your unconscious mind to insert an image on the screen that stands for *yes*. After receiving your *yes* image, blank the screen again. Then ask for a *no* image. This works well for many people, but is not recommended while driving a car!

Pendulums and Dowsing Rods for Muscle Testing

For centuries, people have demonstrated an ability to note the movement of a dowsing rod or pendulum to answer questions intuitively. While initially these were used to locate underground water for wells, their use has broadened to answering the same spectrums of questions as in any other form of muscle testing. It is clear that these are muscle testing devices because when a person's hand is rested on the edge of a table, or when the string is pinched in a vise, the pendulum will not move to answer *yes* or *no* questions.

Dowsing with pendulums and rods extends the use of our unconscious awareness outside of ourselves. This is an intuitive, spiritual use of muscle testing.[5]

Muscle testing can be used as a "truth meter." Having established your *yes* and *no* responses concerning neutral issues, you can proceed to ask yourself questions about your physical or psychological well-being. Simpler questions might concern whether various medicines or other treatment interventions are likely to be helpful, useless, or harmful. You may also explore more complicated questions, such as whether or not it is for your highest good to engage in certain experiences or relationships, or whether unconscious psychological factors could be contributing to a stress state or pain. Any question at all can be posed, as long as they are simplified to allow a *yes* or *no* reply or series of replies.

This was a long introduction to another method for dealing with resistances. When the simpler methods of addressing resistances

---

[5] More on this and related subjects in Chapter 6.

produce no benefits, muscle testing will often open doors to deeper understanding and options we might not have considered otherwise.

Here are generic statements and questions worth checking on one-self with muscle testing when dealing with a resistance. It is often help-ful to ask both of the first two questions, as the second may sometimes be true as well as the first.

- "I am ready to release all of my [issue/pain/stress/belief/disbelief] now."

- "I want [need] to hold onto some of my [issue/pain/stress/belief/dis-belief] now."

- "There are one or more issues from earlier in my life that need clearing in order to release the resistance I am experiencing."

- "My release of this [issue/feeling] is blocked by [issues in my cur-rent relationship with someone else/meta-issues] that make me uncomfortable about releasing this [issue/feeling]."

- "There is/are [one/two/or more] issue(s) from one or more past lives that need(s) clearing in order to release the resistance I am experi-encing."[6]

- "It will be [helpful/necessary] to consult a therapist in order to release my resistance to this issue."

I encourage you to be creative in asking your questions. There are no limits to your inner wisdom. Be sure to record the precise words you use in asking your questions before or as you ask them, so they can be re-evaluated in the light of later analysis. This allows you to tweak the questions for greater clarity and confidence in the answers. Your unconscious mind and higher self are extremely literal and will respond to the exact words you used in framing your questions. If you feel the answers you are getting are too illogical or feel wrong, ask your ques-tion in different ways.

Common pitfalls in muscle testing may include:

- *Neglecting to state a timeframe* — "I will benefit from [WHEE/ Vitamin A/a holiday]" could elicit a *yes* but the benefit might be in ten years. If you want to know about benefits needed *now*, you must specify that.

---

[6] More on clearing past-life issues in Chapter 6.

- *Neglecting to define your terms* — "Will it be good to end this [relationship/work commitment]?" does not specify good for who, good in what way, and (did you catch it?) also *when* to end the relationship. *Good* is a term that also bears clarifying.

- *Overlooking the possibility of several factors being important and relevant simultaneously* — "Will it be good for me to release all of this pain now?" does not contradict the fact that some part of you might still want/feel a need to hold onto some of the pain. It is always helpful to ask the opposite question as well, "Does some part of me want/need to hold onto some of this pain now?" I once also witnessed a *yes* to the second question, but the resistance still didn't release. This person's issue was *fear of releasing the pain*, and his unconscious mind, in its literal way, still said *no* to the second question.

Cautions: One must be extremely careful in interpreting the results of muscle testing. As with any diagnostic procedure (intuitive or physical), there will always be a percentage of false positive and false negative findings. While there is some research to confirm that muscle testing can provide valid answers, as yet, this is very limited. In other words, even under the best of circumstances you will sometimes get wrong answers with muscle testing.

Several ways to reduce the risk of error in muscle testing include:

1. *Use common sense and logical reasoning* to analyze information that arises intuitively. Don't act rashly on the basis of intuitive impressions that contradict reason, and reject intuitive urges that go counter to ethics or moral principles.

2. *Examine your introspective, emotional, and intuitive responses* to the information provided through muscle testing. The information you bring up may be similar to dream imagery, which can be distorted. That is, the *yes* you receive may be a yes to part of a question rather than to the whole question. When in doubt, consult trusted family, friends, and professional therapists.

3. *Reversals* may occur in the muscle testing. Our usual *yes* response may be expressed by the muscles as weakness instead of strength, and our *no* as increased strength. This can happen when we are distressed, ungrounded, in an environment that has dissonant bioenergies, and in other circumstances where we cannot identify the

cause. If you sense that this may be happening, ground yourself again and do some brain balancing exercises. The latter are mostly right and left body stimulation, so you can use any of the WHEE tapping techniques. Massaging the tender spot at the collarbone point also corrects reversals.

4. *Use multiple readings and supplement them with readings by others* —preferably by people such as clinicians who are experienced and expert in the use of these methods—when there are persistent questions and unclarity about results obtained with muscle testing. Similarly, you may hold a question silently in your head and ask a trusted other person to do the muscle testing. This can provide an unbiased *yes* or *no*.

5. *Bioenergies and spiritual connections* can be added to the WHEE procedure to make it more potent, which may also serve to overcome resistances. Coming from the opposite direction, connecting with our intuitive awareness through muscle testing can help to validate our spiritual awareness.[7]

Clearing the Vessel through which Healing Flows

As we clear out and release issues that have been buried, we find that our whole being is clearer of blocks and resistances, starting with our unconscious mind and extending to many other levels. Multiple layers of sweetening spirals are created and facilitated, each of which may be enhanced by the others and may potentiate them, at the same time.

Buried hurts and issues create blocks and resistances to awareness and to flows of energies. If the psychological pain of a loss (e.g. death of someone close/failed relationship/loss of function due to injury or illness) remains buried, the unconscious mind will place sentinels and guards to secure the inner caves where that pain is locked away, hidden from conscious awareness. In its child-like way, the unconscious says, "If we let these painful feelings out, we will only feel the hurt all over again and we might feel just as overwhelmed as we did when we buried them."

---

[7] More on spiritual uses and bioenergies in muscle testing, including further cautions, in Chapters 6 and 7.

The unconscious also says, "Stay away from anything that might rattle the skeletons in that cave." So, we end up avoiding issues that are similar to those we buried in our inner caves. If our buried feelings are those of grief, we will stay away from people and situations that have to do with losses and grief. While this protects us from feeling the buried hurts, it harms us by cutting us off from important slices of human interactions. We cannot keep our cake in the cave and eat it too.

When therapists have buried feelings like these, such as grief or emotional pain of other sorts (some of the most commonly buried issues and feelings), this can be detrimental not only to themselves but to their clients. Therapists can easily divert clients from opening up feelings of grief or pains. This is often a subtle and totally unconscious maneuver on the part of the therapists. They may simply choose to focus on other issues, pushing the ones that are painful to themselves aside.

Therapists' blocks and resistances may thus become a cause of client resistance. The unconscious, Inner Child of clients will readily go along with this resistance, on the childish first principle of avoiding pain. More subtle and pervasive resistances can grow from there, as clients and therapists collude in keeping feelings and issues buried. This strengthens the childhood default of running away from all painful, stressful and unpleasant issues, increasing resistances across the spectrum of whatever issues clients may have buried.

This is why it is important for therapists to have ongoing mentor and/or peer supervision. In such discussions, therapists can explore cases where the resistances are not clearing, and get feedback from others about their own blind spots and resistances.

Psychological resistances often leave us emotionally uptight, which is then reflected in body tensions. Physical and psychological tensions may both contribute to blocks to energy flows. When such blocks are chronic, they can also lead to physical disease. Conversely, when we clear psychological and energetic blocks and resistances, physical problems often clear.

For all of these reasons, I require that therapists who want to take the WHEE Level 2 trainings attend monthly peer supervision meetings. These also expand our understanding of ways that WHEE may or may not be helpful to people in diverse situations and circumstances.

Presence

> *When we honestly ask ourselves which person in our lives means the most to us, we often find that it is those who, instead of giving advice, solutions, or cures, have chosen rather to share our pain and touch our wounds with a warm and tender hand. The friend who can be silent with us in a moment of despair or confusion, who can stay with us in an hour of grief and bereavement, who can tolerate not knowing, not curing, not healing and face with us the reality of our powerlessness, that is a friend who cares.*

> —Henri Nouwen

Much of our experience of pain has to do with our mental and emotional responses to it. We may recall times in the past when we had the same or similar, experience anxieties or fears about the pain continuing or worsening, or worry about the presence or worsening of an associated disease process that is marked by pain. Yet, if we can simply be present with the pain, it will often diminish significantly.

Linda had severe back pain from ruptured disks that had not responded to two surgical interventions over a period of six years. She was unhappy and frustrated with taking the strong pain medications needed to control her pain because she could not find one that did not have unpleasant side effects. She was particularly bothered by mental fuzziness and drowsiness.

Linda was surprised to find that her pain diminished from a 9 to a 6 just by dialoguing with it. This helped her to overcome further skepticism when I suggested that she just hold her awareness of the pain without responding in any way to it. She went very quiet for several minutes. I could see her body relax, her face becoming less taut, and could sense a shift in her energies. Her voice was distinctly softer when she reported with bemusement that her pain had gone down to a 3.

In many cases, using WHEE serves this function of staying present with our pains. In fact, presence is an important components of the WHEE process, in which we do rounds of tapping while focusing on affirmations that acknowledge the presence of the pains.

In my experience of helping many people work through their pain issues, I find that for some, their practice of presence with their physical and psychological pain alone is sufficient. Most, however, find that tapping and affirmations markedly enhance the release of whatever is being invited to let go. You may wish to explore for yourself which components are most helpful, keeping in mind that this may vary with different issues.

If you are a therapist using WHEE or any other modality, you will also find that your presence can be a vital part of the ways you are helpful to your clients. Countless therapists have observed that clients are incredibly grateful just to have someone listen intently to their stories, without their having had to respond verbally or in any other way. Carl Rogers and Eckhart Tolle have developed entire systems of healing based on presence.

It's very easy to feel someone's pain when you love them.

—Salma Hayek

Research on WHEE

I am pleased to share that the first of several studies including WHEE has been completed. Christine Caldwell Bair[8] found that significant synchronizations were demonstrated between heart rates of healer and healee—the primary focus of the study. The volunteer healees came in response to an advertisement to learn a self-relaxation and healing technique that was part of a study. Both the control and treatment groups were also taught WHEE.

Subjects in the treatment group received the WHEE plus a HeartMath-type intervention in which the therapist held the intention to generate greater heartbeat coherence in the subjects of the experiment. This method demonstrated additional significant effects compared to the control group, who only practiced WHEE. Quoting from Bair's doctoral dissertation:

"The objective of this study is to investigate the effect of the healer's heart field upon subjects during energy healing, as measured by synchronization of heart rates and scores on a Subjective Units of Distress (SUD) scale and Profile of Mood States (POMS) inventory.... Statistically significant heart rate synchronization was found in the intervention population. Subjective Units of Distress and Profile

---

[8] See title and web links under References.

of Mood States scores demonstrated more improvement than the control population, indicating additional benefit beyond the WHEE effect alone."

Of note is the demonstration by the control group of a modestly significant decrease in SUDS from their practice of WHEE, which was taught to all 41 participants simultaneously. The researcher also notes in private communications about WHEE: "Anecdotally, I can report that almost all the folks I've had opportunity to teach it to actually *use it* because of it's ease, unobtrusiveness, and effectiveness—very different than other techniques which work fine, but no one uses them because they can't get off alone and find 15-20 minutes to do them, so they just don't bother."

It is helpful to have this objective research confirmation of the efficacy of WHEE. The modality itself is particularly helpful in research because:

- It is easily learned, easy and rapid to use, and very potent and effective.

- WHEE taps into the research database of EMDR and is thus more easily accepted by hospital research boards and conventional medical and nursing researchers and clinicians than many other Energy Psychology modalities. The efficacy of EMDR is gaining acceptance as equivalent to Cognitive Behavioral Therapy for treatment of PTSD by growing numbers of authorities.

Further research is planned, including a study of WHEE for test anxiety in university students.

4

WHEE for Rapid, Deep, and Permanent Pain Relief

The most beautiful people we have known are those who have known defeat, known suffering, known struggle, known loss, and have found their way out of the depths. These people have an appreciation, a sensitivity, and an understanding of life that fills them with compassion, gentleness, and deep, loving concern. Beautiful people do not just happen....

—Elizabeth Kübler-Ross

Although WHEE helps people deal with most pains, it is essential to keep in mind the fact that very different approaches must be used for acute and chronic pains.

Acute pains may come from many of the factors detailed in the first chapter. Such pains are often intense. They may be all the more bothersome because they halt us in our tracks and limit our activities. If we have not had such pains before, they are extra challenging because they are unfamiliar and, therefore, we may not know how to deal with them.

Dealing with Acute Pain

The secret of success is learning how to use pain and pleasure instead of having pain and pleasure use you. If you do that, you're in control of your life. If you don't, life controls you.

—Anthony Robbins

While it may be perfectly obvious that a pain from an accident or surgery is telling us to be careful with that injured part of our body, the pain is nevertheless difficult to deal with.

Explore talking with the pain, and ask what it wants to tell you. When you do this, you may be very surprised in several ways. Most commonly, the pain is saying that it is there to warn you to be gentle with that arm or leg or belly that is hurting. Here are some common comments from a spectrum of pains:

- If it is wound pain: "This is to remind you to be gentle with your wound. It will heal better if you treat me with care and do not re-injure this part of your body."

- If it is a headache, backache, or stomachache that is not due to injury, the message may be more complex. Your pain may speak to you of some sort of disharmony in your life that is making you uptight. Again, your pain is giving a message about treating yourself better. Your pain may be saying, "I'm helping you avoid this situation that is making you uptight," or "This is a sure way to get [your partner/other family member/person at work] to [give you a little more attention/let you off the hook].

Any pain, even from injuries or surgery, may also speak of earlier pains that are stashed away in the same file drawer. I am no longer surprised to see the uncanny abilities of our unconscious mind to invite injuries or create pains internally in order to draw our attention to buried hurts that are now crying to be released. Such pains may be saying, "Please, can't we change these child rules that say we must keep all of these old hurts locked away, and pretend we don't know they are there?"

At the same time, your unconscious mind may be scared to let go of the locks on the filing cabinets and closets and caves where old feelings are stashed. It may be telling you, "Maybe it's not such a good idea to dig around in here!" Such fears may make the pain temporarily worse when we start to work on it.

It is very common to have very rapid, significant decreases in the pain just from the act of dialoguing with it. Your unconscious mind will be most grateful that you—with your adult perspectives, intelligence, and experience—are there to help sort out the tensions and stresses that are leading your unconscious mind to call out to you through these pains.

Different people may experience these sorts of dialogues in other ways. I am used to the term "unconscious mind" and that works for me. Various clients have given this part of themselves a person's name, or identified it as "my wise inner self," "my inner advisor," "my mischief maker," or "my inner policeman." As with any other aspect of WHEE, feel free to connect with the voice inside as it feels right to you to do so.

Next, you can negotiate with the pain, asking it whether it might relent even more if you promise to listen to your unconscious mind whenever it draws your attention by calling out in pain. Your unconscious is really just waiting for you to step in and help it sort out its tensions and conflicts in better ways. Again, this intervention often leads to further decreases in pain.

> Sally, mentioned in the Introduction, had only a limited decrease in her pain through dialoguing with it. It was only when she promised that she would listen faithfully to it when it spoke to her that her pain fully relented.

However, if you do not keep your promises, your pains are likely to return. You may then have a more difficult time convincing your unconscious mind that it could relent and does not have to call your attention to its needs with the pains.

If you do keep your promises, you could then ask your unconscious mind if it would be willing to whisper to you with a gentle ache, rather than screaming at you with pain, when it feels the need to call your attention to a problem. Again, you can expect further decreases in pain.

General Observations About WHEE

It's not what you do but how you do what you do that determines whether you're fulfilling your destiny.

— Eckhart Tolle

Let me digress here briefly. You might be asking, "What does talking with the pain have to do with WHEE?" This is actually very much at the heart of the "W" of WHEE. Wholistic healing addresses the person who has the illness rather than just treating the illness the person has.

If we can help people to identify, understand, and address the underlying issues behind their pain—whether they be recent or old, of physical or psychological origins—then we are sorting out the root causes of the problems. This is ever so much better than taking medications that just dull the symptoms but do not address the underlying causes.

The fact that pains will diminish in response to talking with them is immediate proof that this approach works. People learning to use WHEE are often bemused and surprised when one of my early questions in taking a thorough and detailed history is, "What do you think your pain might be saying to you?" In my experience, about nine out of ten people can quickly find an answer to this question. In fact, it is not uncommon for them to find several meaningful and helpful answers. When they see how quickly their pains respond as they consider their answers to this question, they are then surprised—looking back on months and years of other therapies—that no one had ever asked them this question before.

I suggest that you explore how the various elements of WHEE work for you, in this, as in anything else in this book. By trying on this shoe you will see how it fits. You can know in your innermost being whether what I suggest is true for you. And I encourage you to play with WHEE and tweak it to match your personal preferences, needs and responses.

The next step is to set the stage for using WHEE. After talking with your pain and clarifying how much it may be willing to lighten up just through a dialogue, it is time to negotiate how much it is ready to let go, and whether it might be willing to let go entirely.

With acute pain that has just recently begun to bother you, you can generally expect a willingness to release completely. Chronic pain may or may not be another story.

Start with a dialogue question about how much the pain feels it needs to continue. Sometimes the responses are clear and your course will be obvious. For example:

> I started to feel a tension headache. I was under pressure of several commitments with short deadlines (not unusual for me) and stressed by unexpected client requests for extra sessions. It is rare for me to get headaches, so I stopped to speak with my pain.

It was in the back of my head, extending down my neck. I shook my head in bemusement at not having realized that I chose poorly when I complained about what a "pain in the neck" some of my deadlines were!

My pain relented entirely only when I promised that I would take more frequent breaks from writing and get more sleep.

* * *

Gail, a 24-year-old single graduate student and part-time research assistant, suffered for a year from such intense pre-menstrual pains that she often missed one or two days of work. She was reluctant to take the hormones her doctor prescribed, preferring to address her problems without pills. She had never had counseling or other therapies for this problem, other than massages that relaxed her and enabled her to tolerate the pain better.

In a long dialogue with her pain, Gail discovered that her womb had stored tensions from many issues in her life. Her mother had had similar pains and told her to prepare to suffer when her periods started. An unpleasant abortion during her first year at university had left her very disappointed in her boyfriend, and had resonated with similar feelings of being unsupported by her father. Gail's pains were worsened by stress, particularly when she was under pressures that included evaluations of her work.

Bundling her issues worked well for Gail. In a single WHEE session she was able to reduce her tensions and distressed memories around the pain, and after two months of using WHEE prior to her periods, she was pain free.

Gail had several WHEE sessions that were crucial to her progress between her periods. She needed to work on her pain's worries that if she wasn't careful, she might get close again with a man who would be unsupportive and leave her when she really needed him.

* * *

Fred was an accident-prone 32-year-old teacher. He'd had four fractures in the previous six years from falls in non-contact sports—two riding his bicycle and one each playing baseball and tennis. He came for treatment because his ankle continued to hurt six months after his most recent fracture, well past the time that pain ordinarily ceases with this type of injury.

Dialoguing with his pain, Fred heard that his body did not trust him to be careful with it and was reminding him to not injure himself again. Both Fred and I were surprised at the numbers and varieties of issues that emerged in a series of WHEE sessions from this seemingly simple post-injury pain. Fred had suffered frequent criticisms at times, and at other times neglect from his father and had been pampered by his mother, who was compensating for his father's behaviors. In school, his grades were below average, but he received a lot of praise and attention for his athletic abilities and always pushed himself to perform even better to get more attention and acclaim. In childhood, his mother over-reacted to any illness or injury, even when it was of minor nature. Fred had been divorced a little prior to his first fracture.

Fred used WHEE to address his neediness for attention that was brought to his awareness by the pain, and then cleared a variety of related feelings from his childhood. He was then able to promise his body that he would take better care of it, and would develop better ways for getting attention than through injuries. While his pain did not relent entirely, it was vastly improved fol-lowing his series of WHEE sessions. When he joined a Rotary group and developed other activities and relationships that he felt were nurturing, the pain finally disappeared.

Once we dialogue with our pain, the roots of our feelings that con-tributed to the development of pain will often become obvious. Usually, this awareness is sufficient in itself to release the pain to a large degree, sometimes even entirely. Working with WHEE on the underlying feel-ings will generally release most or all of the remaining pain. When some of the pain lingers, as with Fred's experience, it is usually because our unconscious mind doesn't trust us to keep our promises of changing whatever in our lives has been paining us. When we do actually make the promised changes, the pain will almost always relent at last.

Maintain an open awareness so that you can identify and explore issues and blocks at every level of your being. If we wanted to decrease auto accidents, we would not limit ourselves to being certain that all of the mechanical parts of the car are installed and functioning. We would also address the driver's mental awareness and emotional states, the rules for driving, rewards and punishments for obeying and disobeying the rules, broader issues of courtesy towards others, and people's understandings of the consequences of not paying attention to all of the above. Similarly, in addressing the way we guide ourselves through our life journey in the vehicle we were given at birth, we will do best when we address problems of body, emotions, mind, relationships, and spirit.

Adapting to Chronic Pain

The pain of the mind is worse than the pain of the body.

—Publilius Syrus

When we live with pain over a period of time, we adapt to having this discomfort and the pain becomes an established part of our lives. Much of our accommodation is simple common sense: we learn to not do certain things that may worsen the pain, such as not stressing various muscles and joints when we have arthritis, not eating particular foods when we have irritable bowel syndrome or colitis, or avoiding exposure to drugs that stir allergic reactions.

These shifts in our physical lives often produce secondary shifts in our psychological awareness. We become "that person who has pain." This may seem to be a straightforward fact, but it has enormous varieties of nuances, some of them quite subtle and complex.

Disability

When we are restricted by pain from certain activities, our self-image takes on these limitations as a part of ourselves. People with arthritis move slowly, take care not to bump into things with parts of their bodies that are in pain, are less active and more sedentary. People with frequent migraines live prepared for interruptions in their schedules and plans. People who have fibromyalgia grow to expect others to doubt their word that they are in pain because they have no physical evidence of malfunction of their body and no way to prove they are not faking their pain.

Entitlement and Special Consideration

Pain entitles us to ask for assistance we might otherwise hesitate to request of those around us. This is a particularly transformative hidden benefit of pain for people who are shy or hesitant to ask others for help. Conversely, this may become a crutch that some are reluctant to let go of. Without their pain, they may fear that others will not be there to help them as much.

Pain may be an opportunity for others to give us attention, show us compassion, and lavish their love in ways that they might not demonstrate otherwise. When I went to live in England, I was warned, "England is a place where it's hard to get a kiss off a stiff upper lip." I found that to be very true. People in England are very reserved about showing feelings. Many of them would not openly ask for affection, and consider asking for attention to be shameful. Pain may thus become a doorway for people to invite attention from the one side, and to offer their caring from the other.

Letting go of pain in a culture or family with such restrictions around demonstrating feelings may be a loss that keeps people unconsciously locked into their pains.

Limitations

Pain prevents us from doing certain things. This may be another blessing in disguise. A tension headache may become a convenient excuse for not doing certain chores, for avoiding sexual relations or for not going into a stressful or distasteful work situation.

Suffering

Each difficult moment has the potential to open my eyes and open my heart.

—Myla Kabat-Zinn

People who suffer pains may feel they are being neglected, forgotten, afflicted, or even abused by a higher power. Some may feel that they must have sinned to have "earned" this sort of painful punishment. Others may be carrying specific guilts of commission or omission for which they believe they deserve to be punished.

Some may feel that the burdens they place upon those around them are punishments that these others deserve—for sins of commission or omission on the parts of family members or friends. I am not suggesting that people with pains sit and plot their revenge upon others whom they feel have treated them badly. The inner child, however, may sometimes vent its angers in such ways. These sorts of social pain dynamics are usually completely outside of one's conscious awareness.

All of these are good issues to address with WHEE. I have seen pains markedly lessened when the accompanying sense of suffering is eased.

I have also seen many people enriched through suffering—both their own and the suffering of people close to them. While this is not a path any of us might choose, the challenges entailed in suffering invite us to rise above them. In doing this, we often find resources within ourselves we did not know existed, and deeply meaningful lessons we might never have gained without the suffering.

In rising above suffering, many people connect with their spiritual awareness more deeply. This may include prayers for relief from suffering, opening deep wells of compassion we did not know exist, meeting exceptional healers and teachers, connecting with bioenergies and Gaia energies, and connecting with the Infinite Source.

Compensation

When a person has been in an accident and there is litigation with potentials for monetary compensation, there is a distinct motivation to hold onto their pains. Again, this is usually totally outside of conscious awareness. Nevertheless, compensation for such pain is such a strong motivating factor that many pain therapists will not accept people for treatment until the litigation is settled. Relinquishing pain under such circumstances may prove impossible for many people.

Examples of Chronic Pains Relieved by WHEE

Brenda was a 36-year-old separated high school teacher who had suffered with fibromyalgia for six years. She told a very typical story of having suffered headaches, stomach cramps, loose bowels, weakness, easy fatigability, insomnia, and fuzzy-headedness for two years before a diagnosis was made. Her family and colleagues thought she was just weary from overwork, as she had been incredibly dedicated to inspiring her students to love English Literature, forever seeking new ways to spark their interest and enthusiasm. Brenda's doctor thought she was depressed because her difficult marriage and put her on antidepressants, which numbed her emotions and turned off her sex drive, but did not touch her symptoms.

The fibromyalgia diagnosis was made by a naturopathic physician, who helped with elimination of a Candida yeast infection and the identification of food allergies that were weakening her immune system. Though Brenda's symptoms lightened for a while, they became more severe when her husband left her, largely due to her disinterest in making love.

Referred by a friend, Brenda came with high hopes that WHEE would provide a quick cure to her longstanding difficulties, as her friend had been cured of a phobia and tension headaches in a single session. I explained that her more severe, multiple symptoms might take somewhat longer to deal with, and she seemed willing to explore what WHEE had to offer.

Brenda chose to work first on her insomnia, as she felt that if this piece of her problems improved, then many other pieces would also improve. She found it very encouraging when she was able to return to sleep within minutes, using WHEE, and indeed this did help her have a bit more energy during the day and a little less brain fog. However, WHEE did not seem to be helping when she used it on her headaches, which she found very disappointing, in view of her friend's success with her headaches.

Brenda was slow to connect with the messages her unconscious mind wanted to give her through her bodily symptoms. She also had difficulties in settling into a routine of doing WHEE on her own, even though there was modest progress with her headaches and depression from using WHEE in the therapy sessions.

The breakthrough came when we worked on meta-issues and core beliefs about Brenda's feeling that she had to be there for everyone else's needs, yet had difficulties asking for her own needs to be met. She started to connect with her feelings—both current and from childhood—of hurts and angers over everyone else, such as her four baby brothers and sister and her husband, getting their needs met. She realized that her obsessive nurturing of others allowed her to vicariously enjoy the pleasant feelings they experienced as they were receiving her care.

* * *

Sal had been healthy and strong all of his life, having seen doctors only for stitches and broken bones from injuries in his construction work and an auto accident. At 52, he was happy in his work, marriage, and role as weekend "spoiler" for four grand-children. He was a stoic man of few words and rarely complained about his health, even when he was slowed down by occasional injuries. His stoicism may have contributed to the late diagnosis of cancer in his esophagus, which had spread to many lymph nodes by the time he finally went to the doctor because of severe pains in his back. X-rays showed metastases in his lower spine

Sal was started on chemotherapy and radiotherapy, which he tolerated poorly. He had headaches and nausea and became depressed and withdrawn. The pain medication made him grog-gy and drowsy (on top of his chemo- and radiotherapy, which also made him tired), and he couldn't even enjoy a football game on TV without dozing off. Sleeping during the day left him wide awake at times during the night. When his doctor prescribed a sleeping pill, he rebelled. Betty, his wife, called me after an Internet search, asking if there was anything WHEE could offer her husband.

I worked with Sal over the phone. He was aware that he had little time left to live, and was willing to work with WHEE on the hopes that he would be less of a burden on his family and able to enjoy watching the Dolphins on their winning streak.

WHEE was very effective in reducing Sal's back pain to levels where he needed much less pain medication and was then more clear-headed. WHEE also reduced his headaches and nausea with chemotherapy.

Despite his stoicism, Sal was a sensitive man. He silently struggled with his grief over the short time he had left to live. Just being able to speak with someone over the phone was a big relief to him, as he feared he would upset his family if he spoke with them of these issues. WHEE helped him release these fears, which also stirred memories from when he had been eight years old and his parents held back their feelings when his father was robbed and severely beaten, suffering severe brain injury. Sal cried more with me over his feelings about his father than he did about himself.

I encouraged Sal to speak with Betty, and they both reported feeling ever so much closer as a result of these conversations.

I had a warm thank-you note from Betty several months later, reporting that Sal had been able to find much more peace and enjoyment in his last six weeks. He had even found the strength to say his farewells to his children and grandchildren. Betty was very appreciative and grateful for the help they had received, which she felt had brought their family much closer together.

Dialoguing with Chronic Pain

You will not grow if you sit in a beautiful flower garden,

but you will grow if you are sick, if you are in pain, if you experience losses,

and if you do not put your head in the sand,

but take the pain and learn to accept it,

not as a curse or a punishment

but as a gift to you with a very, very specific purpose.

—Elizabeth Kübler-Ross

Although we have already addressed dialoguing with pain in some detail, this subject deserves a separate discussion of its own with respect to chronic pain. Many people who have come to me for help with long-term issues have been astounded at the simple suggestion that they talk with their pain. Oftentimes I am the first to have ever recommended this simple approach, even after many years of seeking pain relief through enormous ranges and varieties of methods. Still, about 9 out of 10 people can immediately begin to find helpful, often deeply meaningful responses to the questions they ask their pains.

When dealing with chronic pain it can be especially helpful to have the guidance of a therapist in this dialogue process, as the issues themselves are often deeply imbedded, multi-layered, and completely outside of conscious awareness. The responses we receive depend very much on the questions we ask and how we conceptualize and phrase them. As with our phrasings of the affirmations for WHEE, we must always remember that the unconscious mind is extremely literal and will answer with great precision the specific questions we have asked.

Wanda was a married, 48-year-old teacher who suffered from severe tension headaches. She learned quickly to lower the intensity of the headaches from a SUDS of 9 or 10, but could not get the pain to reduce below a 5 or 6.

Wanda was in a marriage that she found unsatisfying in many ways. Her husband, Larry, earned a good living and they were able to enjoy the benefits of a very comfortable lifestyle. She admitted that this was a major reason for her decision to stay in the relationship, even though she and her husband had grown apart as he became increasingly interested in spectator sports and they did less and less together as a couple.

With direction and encouragement, Wanda was able to use WHEE to overcome her anxieties and confronted Larry with her unhappiness about their drifting apart. To her surprise and relief, he responded with concern and caring, and their relationship started to improve.

Disappointingly, her headaches went down only to an intensity of 3 or 4. This appeared to be connected with Wanda's continued dissatisfaction with Larry, which both she and I agreed seemed to be excessively strong in view of the promisingly good start at improvements, her earlier good relationship with him, and her positive feelings and wishes for making the relationship work.

This suggested to me that there might be other issues sitting in Wanda's file drawer that resonated with her current issue. Wanda asked her pain if it was holding on because of experiences with someone in the past who had resembled her husband, and the answer was a clear no. Knowing her history of having had an unhappy relationship with her father throughout her childhood, I encouraged Wanda to ask the question in a different way. When she drew a blank, I suggested she ask, "Are there leftovers from my childhood relationship with my father that are getting in the way of my relationship with Larry?" The answer was a clear yes.

Working on these issues was the key to releasing the pain entirely. Wanda's unconscious mind was ready and eager to have her clear these old issues. One might even speculate whether she hadn't chosen Larry as her partner in life out of this inner wish/need to clear these issues.

I encourage people to use WHEE for clearing their own issues at home between therapy sessions. In most cases this is a very positive, successful experience. However, there are times when a person may not be able to identify what issues need exploring and releasing. A part of the problem here is that the issues have been long buried by the unconscious mind—either because they were overwhelmingly uncomfortable or simply out of the default habit of burying issues that are bothersome. In either case, it may be difficult for a person to connect with the issues that are causing their problems. An outside party who does not share the same problems may be able to help identify the relevant issues. This is an example of why therapists need to work on themselves to "clear the vessel through which healing flows."

Here is another example of the need for clarity in dialoguing with the unconscious mind about pain:

Joe was a 32-year-old department store salesman. He came to me for help with chronic backaches that had plagued him for more than 20 years and worsened in the past three. Joe was a caring, gentle person who was eager to learn to help himself, despite difficulties in expressing his feelings, as this was not something he had ever done before. Repeated medical examinations had shown no physical cause for the pain, and chiropractic adjustments provided only partial, temporary relief, never lasting more than two to three days.

Dialoguing with his pain, Joe found that it was helping him to be aware of stresses in his life that he otherwise tended to ignore. These included a domineering wife and excessive demands from his employers to put in overtime. Working with WHEE on these stresses and on Joe's hesitations to stand up for himself brought the pains down from a SUDS of 6 to 8 to a much more tolerable level of 3 or 4. However, he could not get the pain to relent further, despite clearing the above and other issues in his current life that contributed to the pain.

It felt likely to me that there were other issues sitting in Joe's file drawer that had not yet surfaced. I explained to him that some traumatic experience could have been buried by his unconscious mind, due to childhood programming. So, Joe began another dialogue with his pain. He asked, "Is there an event in my file drawer from the past that is causing you to persist?" The answer was "no." We checked with muscle testing, and the answer was the same, though I thought I detected a slight, subtle difference between this no by muscle testing and other no responses from the past.

I encouraged Joe to ask other questions, but he could not think of anything to ask. So I suggested that he ask if there was a reason to not reveal the reason. To his surprise, there was a strong yes response.

Long story short, through further explorations and work with WHEE Joe was able to uncover memories of being sodomized by an older cousin who was baby sitting him when Joe was 12 years old—just prior to the onset of his back pains. The fact that his unconscious had been unwilling to even acknowledge the presence of this event as a contributor to the back pain had to do with several different meta-issues. Joe had been raised in a refugee family from South America that was very strict about not talking with anyone outside the family about family business. In addition, his favorite aunt, the mother of the cousin who sodomized him, had fragile diabetes and Joe was afraid of upsetting her if he revealed what her son had done.

His unconscious mind responded "no" to his question about an issue from the past causing the pain because it was not the incident that was frustrating him so much as it was his sense of injustice in what had happened to him, struggles with the family rules about silence with "outsiders," and his concern about his aunt's health that were making him uptight.

The rules by which we play the game of life are often programmed into our unconscious mind when we are too young to evaluate whether they are in our best interests. When we work on identifying and clearing buried issues, these inner rules may block our awareness and raise resistances. The rules themselves can be very difficult for people to identify because they have been so much a part of us, for so long, that they are perceived and experienced as our natural way of being in the world. It may take a skilled therapist to help to sleuth out these rules that create blocks to release. With its emphasis on muscle testing and rapid releases of limiting rules and beliefs, WHEE is particularly helpful with such resistances.

Life is the only game in which the object of the game is to learn the rules.

—Ashleigh Brilliant

Gently and Slowly Lightening the Burden of Chronic Pain

Considering all of the above ways in which people change as they accommodate their lives to living with chronic pains, it may come as no surprise to you that it may sometimes be best to relieve long-standing pain slowly and gradually. This is particularly true of methods such as WHEE, which may actually be too effective for some people with chronic pains, who can be can traumatized or at least seriously unsettled when too much pain is released at once. This may seem counterintuitive, but it is not unlike putting on a new shoe after wearing the same old, unsupportive pair for a very long time: It looks good and may feel reasonably okay at first, but very quickly it begins to rub here and there. Only once the shoe has been broken in do we feel comfortable walking around in it. This is why I recommend that chronic pain be released a few steps at a time, even though it may be possible in many cases to relieve it entirely in one series of WHEE.

Muscle testing can be enormously helpful in determining how slowly or quickly to release chronic pains. People are very often surprised to find their muscles going weak when they say, "I am fully ready to release all of this pain forever, *now*," or when their muscles remain strong when they say, "I need to hold onto some of this pain now."

There is no need for embarrassment or distress about your unconscious mind feeling it is not ready to let go completely of the lifestyle and psychological habits developed in adjusting to living with pain. These habits were not created overnight. They may have been built up through many months and years of suffering. Releasing them too quickly could be a shock to your system.

The handy thing about WHEE is that it invites you to explore the reasons for any resistances and offers you a variety of ways to work on these as well as on the pain. But here, too, I urge you to move gradually and not to rush. If you find, for instance, that your pain has provided a currency for exchanging caring between you and your family or friends, start looking for ways you could invite a show of caring other than through pain. Once you have some new ways to invite people to demonstrate their caring for you, you can then address the old habits and beliefs around using pain to invite others to offer you their love. You may do well to discuss these issues with those who have been there for you in caring manners. Once you are clear about this and have started to develop new ways of asking for and demonstrating caring, then you will find it most helpful to use WHEE further to dismantle old anxieties and beliefs about how you ask for a show of love.

As we address the ways pain has come to benefit us in our lives, we often become aware of meta-anxieties we have developed. Common examples of these include:

- If I didn't have pain no one would [help/be there for] me.

- If I didn't have pain, I wouldn't know how to ask for [help/caring/love].

- If I ask for attention I won't be [heard/accepted/satisfied].

- My [mother/father] wasn't able to respond to my needs, so no one else can be expected to do so, either.

Similar to meta-anxieties, but deeper in their origins and with more pervasive effects in our lives, are what I call *core beliefs*. Common core beliefs relevant to relinquishing pain may include:

- I'm not worthy of being loved.

- I don't deserve to be loved because...

- Since my [mother/father/other caregiver] didn't love me, nobody will love me.

- If I allow myself to feel loved openly, I will release all the buried hurts from times when I didn't feel loved.

Core beliefs, just like meta-anxieties, can be addressed with WHEE by assessing the cognitions (such as those listed above) for their SUDS levels then decreasing their intensity to zero using the same process as with feeling issues. At that point, a positive replacement cognition (opposite to the negative cognition that was released) can be installed. For instance, one could work on "Even though I believe I'm not worthy of being loved," adding as one alternates tapping each side of the body, "I still love and accept myself..." When the SUDS is down to zero, one would carefully craft a positive replacement, such as, "I am fully worthy of being loved..." or, "As a child of God, I..." then round this out with an affirmation positive, such as "love and accept myself, wholly and completely."

Once the core belief has been released, it is helpful to ask with muscle testing whether this is sufficient so that your [inner self/higher self/whole being/however you conceptualize your unconscious mind] is comfortable with proceeding now to work further on your pain directly using WHEE.

A second good question to ask with muscle testing is whether it might be [for your highest good/helpful to you and those who are close with you] to take a break from working on your pain with WHEE. Keeping the pace gradual may allow time for you who are experiencing the pain—and for everyone else who is involved in your circle of relationships—to adjust to less pain in their lives.

Keep in mind, though, that muscle testing might reveal affirmative answers to *both* of these last questions! You might then make your decision based on your own conscious assessment of your situation, in consultation with those who have been helping you with your pain, and/or by further clarifying through muscle testing or dialoguing with your pain. Multiple inputs are highly advisable in making such decisions. When we rely on our own awareness, either conscious or unconscious, we may sometimes be disappointed in the outcomes of our decisions. It is very easy to be over-focused on one aspect of the issue we are addressing and to overlook other elements. When this is the case, the decisions we make will be valid for the specific questions we are posing, but the questions themselves may be too narrow, out of focus, or off target in regards to important aspects of our lives that we are not taking into consideration at that moment.

Susie was a cute, outgoing eight-year-old tomboy who had suffered from arthritis for a year following a bout of rheumatic fever. The pains in her knees had been so severe that she was actually bedridden twice for several weeks at a time. Her parents were unhappy with her having to take many medications, some of which made her groggy, while others had potentially dangerous side effects. Fortunately, WHEE was rapidly effective in reducing her pains from a SUDS of 7 or 8 down to 2 or 3.

Still, Susie was frustrated and angry when her pains did not clear entirely. I cautioned her and her family to go slowly with WHEE, explaining that the pain was a reminder to her to not run around and stir up the arthritis in her knees, which would then prolong her suffering.

As she improved, she began to be oppositional and rebellious around doing chores and schoolwork, and her parents realized just how much they had tended to her needs. In simple language, she had been spoiled through the necessary pampering she received while debilitated. As they sorted out these issues, Susie, her two older sisters, and her parents all benefited from using WHEE.

* * *

Darryl was a married 45-year-old truck driver who had suffered severe backaches for 15 years following an accident at work. He was very unhappy with the fogginess he experienced when he took powerful pain medicines, and equally unhappy when he reduced his medication and suffered more from the backaches.

Darryl found WHEE helpful in reducing his pain from a SUDS of 9 or 10 down to 7 or 8. By addressing meta-anxieties and core beliefs he succeeded in lowering it even more, to a 6. He was disappointed, however, when he could not lower the pain further, even though his muscle testing indicated that all of his being was ready to do so.

I encouraged Darryl to enjoy his lesser levels of pain for a week, observing where there might still be reasons to hold onto it, and recommended strongly that he not rush to reduce it further at that time, and certainly not to eliminate it completely.

At his next session, Darryl reported he had discussed his decreased pain with his wife, Zena. They had come to understand that if and when his pain was completely gone, this could bring about major changes in their lives on many, many levels. She was particularly looking forward to being able to take walks with him in nature again, as she missed his company a lot but had done this on her own rather than not do it at all. Still, she felt that the pain, overall, had brought them closer together, as he had not been going out with the guys as much. She was concerned that he might go back to spending time at the bar after work and attending hockey games, to the detriment of the closeness they had developed. She also pointed out that he would be able to do many chores he had been unable to muster himself to do for years. (Darryl was actually taken aback a bit by this response, as he hadn't realized the burden that Zena had gradually taken on as he became less and less able to help around the house.)

With little urging on my part, Darryl readily agreed to go slowly with further pain reductions, so that he and Zena had time to adjust to the changes this could bring to their relationship. He actually found that he enjoyed her company more than that of the crowd at the bar—which was a big relief to Zena. They had also discussed which chores he might pick up on first. And so his return to more normal life activities was gradually sorted out, with periodic uses of WHEE for acute pain control and then further decreases in pain.

* * *

Jeff was a warm but stoic 66-year-old retired nurse who came to me for help with pain from pancreatic cancer he had struggled with for six months. He readily reported that he was better at helping others than he was at asking for help for himself. His wife, Anna, confirmed this and added that she was more than ready to care for Jeff in any way she could, but that she had found it difficult throughout their marriage to know when or how to demonstrate her love for him because he was so was so quick to say, "It's all right. I can handle this myself." Now that he was weak, not only from the cancer but also from the chemotherapy and radiotherapy for his primary lesion and metastases, Anna dearly wanted to pamper him—but he was not letting her get closer.

In dialoguing with his SUDS level-9 pain, Jeff learned that his Inner Child really was crying out for more tenderness and nurturing. WHEE was helpful to him in lightening up on his core belief that he had to handle things for himself—which had stood him in good stead during his difficult childhood in an orphanage. Both Jeff of today and Little Jeff, however, could readily see that this belief was no longer appropriate, and were happy to release it with WHEE.

Jeff's pain, however, remained unchanged. In further dialogue, Jeff's pain said that his Inner Child did not trust him to keep his word to ask Anna for attention, and therefore was reluctant to lower the intensity of pain. When Jeff promised that he would actually practice asking for help, his pain relented and dropped down to a SUDS of 2 with a few rounds of WHEE.

Dealing with meta-anxieties and core beliefs can sometimes be a challenge. We are so used to our habitual ways of perceiving and responding to the world that we may have difficulties identifying where we are hung up with our affirmations. The help of a professional counselor, family members, and friends who can coach us to clarify our issues may markedly facilitate the effectiveness of WHEE.

The above examples help to illustrate these points. Jeff's experiences also illustrate how pain may be present, at least in part, to motivate a person to do or not do certain things. It is often easy to get one's pains to lessen by negotiating with them. I have many times seen pain respond to a request combined with a promise: "If I keep my word and [move about with care not to stress or re-injure myself/ask for help when I am feeling in need of attention/follow my self-care routines faithfully] then would you please whisper to me with pain instead of shouting at me?"

One of the most helpful aspects of WHEE is that it can be focused on any level of issue or resistance. As soon as progress is blocked, the meta-anxiety, belief, or disbelief that is holding a person back from releasing the issue can be identified and dealt with through WHEE.

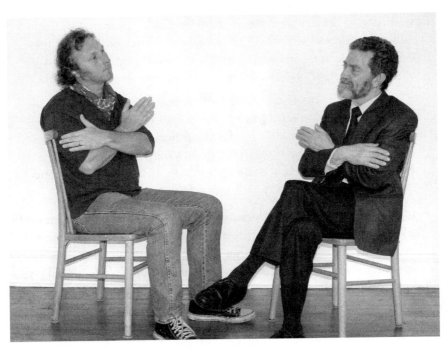
Dr. Benor teaching WHEE.

5

The Unconscious Mind and WHEE

The Unconscious is not unconscious, only the Conscious is unconscious of what the Unconscious is conscious of.

—Francis Jeffrey

While we have seen many ways in which the unconscious mind can participate in our WHEE healings, it is well worthwhile to discuss this particular topic as a separate focus. The unconscious mind is a vast resource that we can tap into for our benefit. It is estimated to contain 95 percent of all that we know. It serves as integrator for new awareness and learning, control system for our bodily functions, memory bank, automatic pilot for habitual behaviors, channel for intuitive/psychic awareness, link with our higher self, and more.

Integrator for New Awareness and Learning

Just when you think you've graduated from the school of experience, someone thinks up a new course.

—Mary H. Waldrip

A newborn infant does not appear to have the abilities to integrate and interpret sensory inputs. For example, it takes several months for a baby's eyes to focus on an object. The first thing a baby comes to recognize is almost always its mother's face. In part, this appears to be a genetic imprint, as a baby will respond to a sketchy picture of eyes, nose, and mouth on a sheet of paper, tracking it with its eyes and smiling before it will track and respond to other objects.

The brain is an enormously complex organ, containing an estimated one hundred billion neurons (nerve cells). Neurons in the brain communicate through electrical and chemical signals with many thousands of other nerve cells in the spinal cord and in networks extending throughout the body. In this way, information is brought into the brain and messages are sent to the body to regulate its musculoskeletal actions and organ functions.

Some of the controls of the nervous system—such as heart rate, respiration, and digestion—develop automatically and are generally involuntary and unconscious. Other functions, such as control of musculoskeletal movements, are learned through both conscious and unconscious feedback loops. A simple example of this is when a child learns to bring a bit of food with her hand to her mouth. Through a complex process of inputs—including visual, touch, and kinesthetic sensations—combined with the reward of a good taste, with multiple trials for successes and errors the brain learns to interpret all of these inputs and to control the muscles so that food can be regularly and reliably brought to her mouth. You may recall in later life the similar processes of learning to ride a bicycle or drive a car. At first, you have to pay attention to each and every movement and may be clumsy and have to repeat your movements many times to get them right.

Functional Control Systems

Much illness is unhappiness sailing under a physiologic flag.

—Rudolf Virchow

The unconscious mind controls bodily functions of many sorts, on varieties of levels. We are at least subconsciously aware of our control over the muscles we activate at will—to lift a cup for a sip of tea, for example, or to scan our eyes across the pages of this book. We usually have no awareness, however, of our automated bodily controls, such as those over the secretion of gastric juices and contractions of intestinal muscles that move our lunch along its way through the digestive system, or the rhythms of heartbeats, blood pressure, and muscles that move air in and out of our lungs at varying rates. Nor are we conscious of the biochemical feedback systems that regulate these body functions. For instance, as our muscles produce carbon dioxide in exertion and require more oxygen, the chemical composition of our blood will also influence our heartbeats, blood pressure, and breathing...all without our ever thinking about it.

Modern science has developed ways to alert us to our own levels of blood pressure and heartbeats. When we have this sort of biofeedback, we may develop conscious controls over these functions. You can demonstrate this for yourself:

- With a finger on the pulse of your wrist, you can learn to slow or speed up your heart rate.

- Learn to contract the iris of your eye at will by practicing with visual feedback while looking in a mirror. This can take an hour, on average. (When I read about this as a teenager, I learned to wiggle my ears with mirror biofeedback. I don't recall how long this took.)

Interestingly, as far as internal mechanisms are concerned, no one can tell you how to learn to achieve these controls over muscles that are ordinarily on automatic pilot. You have to experiment for yourself to discover the inner connections that will work for you.

More than just parlor tricks, conscious ability to manipulate otherwise automated controls can be greatly beneficial to our health and well-being. Science now understands how stress can raise blood pressure, tighten arteries that cause migraine headaches, and tighten muscles that give us tension headaches and other pains. Through biofeedback we can learn to alter many of the functions of our body to correct these unwanted responses that contribute to or cause distress or illnesses.

The Mind and the Immune System

Our cells are constantly eavesdropping on our thoughts and being changed by them. A bout of depression can wreak havoc with the immune system; falling in love can boost it.

— Deepak Chopra

Our brain cells contain more than 50 different proteins called neuropeptides, which are active in chemical communications between nerve cells. The very same neuropeptides are also found in the white cells of our immune system. It is presumed that this enables communications between our brain and immune systems. This may explain how the mind can contribute to the development of immune problems such as arthritis, fibromyalgia, cancer, and AIDS. Conversely, it may also explain how the mind can help to relieve or even reverse the courses of these illnesses.

Psychoneuroimmunology (PNI)—which includes varieties of approaches such as relaxation, meditation, imagery (of strengthening the immune system) and support groups—has been shown to be effective for dealing with conditions of immune system malfunction. For instance, it has helped people with cancer to live longer, and in some cases appears to have halted or even reversed the progress of cancer growth by enhancing the activity of their immune system.

Unfortunately, many people seek help from PNI and other complementary/alternative medical (CAM) therapies only late in their course of illness, when all conventional therapies have been exhausted. By that time, many of the body's natural resources for dealing with illness have usually been exhausted and CAM interventions can only be of limited help.

WHEE can provide strong support to the immune system through relaxation and release of stress—both from current problems and issues carried in the unconscious from the past. I have seen excellent results with WHEE in arthritis, not just in reducing pain but also in decreasing swelling and increasing range of motion of joints. Arthritis is presumed to be a disorder in which the immune system attacks the body's own connective tissues, for reasons that are as yet not fully explained.

> At a WHEE workshop in Mexico, a woman with arthritis in her hands volunteered in front of the group to explore how WHEE might help her pain. She had not been able to bend any of her fingers for many months due to modest swelling and severe pain. We did an experiment, having her focus the WHEE on one finger. Within minutes, she was able to bend that finger without pain, but not any of her other fingers.

I have seen numbers of other people with arthritis show significant improvements with WHEE. Commonly, WHEE can also help with psychological issues that are associated with the arthritis, including frustration, anger, depression, and other issues. This is particularly promising, as I find that anger is often a contributing factor to the development and persistence of the arthritis and not just a reaction to its presence.

Another apparent autoimmune disorder that has been shown to be positively affected by WHEE is fibromyalgia, in which people suffer from total fatigue and weakness, tiredness, muscle aches in many parts of their bodies, headaches, "brain fog" (mental fuzziness and confusion), insomnia, and multiple allergies to foods and other substances. WHEE has been helpful to people with fibromyalgia for treating pains and insomnia, for de-stressing for clearing allergies;for addressing old, buried, traumatic issues and transforming self-defeating beliefs that are common with this disorder, as detailed in the story of Brenda, in Chapter 3.

Automatic Pilot for Habitual
Behaviors and Psychological Responses

> *Your actions become your habits*
>
> *Your habits become your values*
>
> *Your values become your destiny.*

—Mahatma Gandhi

With practice, your movements in habitual behaviors become automatic. Take driving, for example: You no longer have to think about each and every reaction in response to road challenges. You may even find at times that you have driven for many minutes, over many miles without conscious awareness of having controlled your car. Yet the evidence is obvious that your unconscious mind navigated the distance without problems.

In a similar manner, your emotional responses become habits. If you grow up in a calm atmosphere at home, your nervous system usually becomes set to automatic calmness in ordinary situations. If your home is a place that has a lot of tensions and stormy emotions, your nervous system may be set to automatic physical and psychological tensions in ordinary situations. There may also be specific stimuli that set off stronger reactions, such as excessive tensions when someone in your current life is angry—whether or not the anger is directed toward you.

Your beliefs about the world may have been strongly colored by your life experiences. It is not uncommon for people to have self-doubts or limiting beliefs that seriously taint or even cripple their enjoyment of life. You also have meta-beliefs and core beliefs, which are more general rules about your place in the world, such as:

- I don't deserve to be loved.

- I will never succeed at anything, so it's no use trying.

- I'm stupid/dumb/a hopeless case/bad.

- I doomed to follow in my mother's/father's footsteps/patterns.

WHEE is wonderful for reprogramming such habitual psychological beliefs, along with the physical reactions that accompany them. People regularly report that tensions in their chest, stomach, back, neck, or other parts of their bodies are released as they use WHEE to let go of their negative psychological responses.

Memory Banks

A remembered stress, which is only a wisp of thought, releases the same flood of destructive hormones as the stress itself.

—Deepak Chopra

Conventional science and medicine view the brain as the storage vault for most of our life experiences.. As evidence for this theory they cite the fact that when portions of the brain are destroyed by injury, disease, or surgery, portions of memory are lost. My understanding of these processes, based on research in spiritual dimensions[1], is that the brain is like a radio or TV receiver that channels your mind and translates the consciousness of spirit and soul into the physical dimension.

Regardless of the mechanism, which cannot be proved in any way that we have yet discovered, our unconscious mind stores enormous numbers of detailed memories of almost everything we experience. It has been amply demonstrated under hypnosis that we can recall tiny details from our childhood that in some cases can be verified. For instance, one woman in her forties described the wallpaper design in the room she slept in as an infant. The hypnotist visited the woman's

---

[1] These studies are thoroughly reviewed in *Healing Research, Volume 3.*

former home, which was still standing, and was able to peel back layers of wallpaper until he uncovered the precise design she had described.

In addition to our own personal memories from throughout our current lives, we may also have memories of past lives. If this sounds unreasonable or unlikely to you, I cannot blame you. For many years, I too was a firm disbeliever in reincarnation. I thought it was either just the wishful thinking of individuals who were afraid of dying, or a collective wish with the same motives that had coalesced into a religious teaching in certain cultures, over long periods of time. However, as we will discuss in the section on reincarnation memories and WHEE in Chapter 6, it appears that the topic deserves serious consideration.

Channel for Intuitive/Psychic Awareness

Letting go of the need to always understand is one of the most powerful steps toward living a soulful life. Moving from know-it-all to spiritual trust is the bridge that carries you into soulful spirituality.

—Bradford Keeney

Most of us have experienced one or more types of intuitive awareness.

Pattern recognition is demonstrated when you have seen many varieties of dogs and a completely new type walks by that you have never seen before. Your unconscious mind identifies the new animal as a dog. This is better than any ordinary computer can do, because computers recognize specific images they have identified previously, but not new ones.

Pattern recognition is extremely helpful to experienced therapists. As I have seen hundreds of people who released buried issues from the file drawers in their unconscious minds, this makes it much easier for me to help new clients identify similar buried issues that are resonating with current problems. The patterns of anxieties that are resisting release have a similar intuitive feel to them. It is difficult to describe this to other therapists who have not had similar experiences.

Extrasensory Perception (ESP), also called *psi* (after the Greek letter Ψ), can help us identify what is happening beyond our physical selves in a variety of ways: *Telepathy* is the ability to read the thoughts of another person. *Clairsentience* is the direct awareness of the condition of an organism or object outside ourselves. For instance, we may intuitively know that a lost object or person is located in a particular place. *Precognition* and *retrocognition* are the perceptions of events that occurred in the past or future. These intuitive perceptions may occur unbidden, spontaneously, or may be intentionally invited by people who are naturally gifted or who have developed their intuitive abilities deliberately.

Many would designate these abilities as being in spiritual dimensions (and therefore more appropriate for discussion in Chapter 6). I believe, however, that these abilities are so intrinsically a part of our unconscious, intuitive processes that they belong in this basic discussion on the functions of our minds. In addition, these aspects of intuition connect us also with spiritual awareness, and will be discussed further in the next chapter.

ESP can be enormously helpful in assisting people to resolve their pains and other problems. Spiritual healers and medical intuitives may be able to sense what is happening in a person's body, emotions, mind, relationships, and spirit. This can be helpful in identifying issues that are producing or contributing to resistances.

While the help of an outside intuitive can be an enormous boost, it may also be disempowering. When an outsider provides answers to challenging questions and recommends ways to address resistances, people may come to rely on the outsider to poke about in the file drawers and caves of their unconscious mind, rather than learning to do this themselves. Also, intuitives do not read a person like a book. Rather, intuitives seem to peer into a window of limited scope within a person. Different intuitives will have views through different windows. Only we, ourselves, can determine what is truly relevant to the analysis of our issues. I believe that our own introspections and explorations of our own unconscious are likely to produce the most valid answers to questions about our pains and other issues. Having said this, I have to add that not everyone has abilities to look inward for themselves. There is definitely a place for outside help from medical intuitives and healers.

Muscle testing can be used to access our own ESP. Since the unconscious mind can give *yes* or *no* answers to our questions, this method allows us to ask questions about issues beyond our ordinary sensory knowledge. These inner, intuitive explorations can then enhance our confidence in our too-often neglected intuitive senses. I encourage people to start with playful experiments such as the following:

When you are shopping for fruits and vegetables, ask your higher self, "Is this [canteloupe/avocado/watermelon/or so forth] going to be fully ripe and tasty on [insert date required]?"

When you are approaching a red light, ask, "Which lane will be best to wait in?" Be clear what you mean by *best*. You may be thinking only that best equals fastest travel across the intersection, but best as in *for your highest good* might be to go more slowly and avoid a traffic accident at the intersection or later along your way.

If you are a therapist, you might ask for *yes* and *no* answers to questions about helping your client. I often have intuitive awareness during therapy and ask my higher self, using unobtrusive muscle testing on myself, "Is this information for this client's highest good to know now?" As often as not, the information is for me rather than for the clients, to help me understand and better assist the clients to help themselves.

Again, you will enhance your appreciation and understanding of these valuable aspects of your unconscious mind by journaling your intuitive impressions—and the feedback you get from life experiences regarding how helpful/valid they are (or are not).

Going further with our intuitive abilities, not only is our consciousness able to connect with the world outside ourselves in exchanges of information, but it is also able to influence the world directly through our wishes, intents, or prayers.

Wakening to Shadow Aspects of Ourselves

If you bring forth what is within you, what you bring forth will save you. If you do not bring forth what is within you, what you do not bring forth will destroy you.

— The Gospel of Thomas

In Jungian psychology, and now in more popular usage, those parts of ourselves that we have shut off from conscious awareness are called our *shadow*. While the unconscious mind is the cave where we hide those feelings and memories we would rather not deal with, it is also a part of ourselves that knows we can do better than following the child programs of burying and running away from the unpleasant item. So the unconscious protects us dutifully, as it has been programmed to do, but still looks for ways to waken us to better options.

Pain is one of the manners in which the unconscious mind speaks about disharmonies in our lives and complains about overloads of emotions and buried materials that the unconscious feels we could deal with in better ways. From the examples of dialogues with pain earlier in this book, you can see that many pains are invitations to release buried feelings and tensions. As soon as we listen to our unconscious mind's alarm bells of pain, our pains can be lessened. Simply by acknowledging that the pain has gotten our attention, we will often find our pains decreased. After negotiating with the pain and promising to attend to the underlying issues, we can then use WHEE to lessen the pain even more, sometimes even eliminating it.

Another way in which the unconscious calls for our attention is to whisper to us through our dreams or to shout and scream at us with nightmares. Dreams are wonderful windows into our being. Every element in a dream is a symbolic part of ourselves wanting our attention. There are countless layers to our dreams. After dialoguing with them to discern their messages and meanings, we can often use WHEE for clearing those issues from our shadow that the dreams bring to our conscious awareness.

Trudy was happy to be moving from San Francisco to New York for a new job with lots of promise for career advancement. She had friends and relatives in New York and was even gifted with a temporary apartment-sitting opportunity that would ease her transition.

Several weeks prior to her move, she was surprised to waken with a distressing nightmare in which she lost all her belongings in the move and ended up in a sleazy New York motel, penniless and friendless. Having had experience in long-term therapy and knowing WHEE, Trudy dialogued with the Trudy of her dream. She uncovered memories of a series of moves during her childhood, after her mother abruptly left her father due to his verbal and physical abuse, when they had ended up in the sort of situation depicted in her nightmare. Using WHEE, she cleared the residues that her unconscious mind had invited her to release from the caves where they had been buried when they were too painful for eight-year-old Trudy to bear.

Dreams are marvelous invitations to housecleaning with WHEE. Through dialoging with elements in our dreams we can often understand the underlying issues asking to be cleared. Furthermore, when these are not evident we can invite any of the characters in our dreams to use WHEE on their own distressing feelings. The images in our dreams will connect with whatever issues have come together to create them, so the WHEE will go where it is needed. This can be especially helpful to children who may not identify exactly what has upset them but can readily use WHEE to deal with a monster that has frightened them in their nightmare.[2]

Switchboard/Control Panel for
Collective Consciousness and Manifestations of Soul

Experiences manifested in your life by the resistance you still possess are there in the interest of truth and light. They show you the pain of these obstructions so you can move through them. In the faith of knowing that all things are moving toward God, the obstructions take on a different meaning and form: they are there at the human level to obstruct; but at the ultimate level to instruct.

—Emmanuel

The unconscious mind constantly seeks ways to waken us on all levels of our being. It is aware of our participation in the collective consciousness and the Infinite Source. It will invite us to connect more consciously with our broader participations in reality, to the extent that we are ready to go there.

As we release our fears of relating to the physical world in more open ways, we become more open as well to connecting more fully and more consciously with our spiritual selves. Pain can be a wonder-full stimulus to facilitate these connections.[3]

---

[2] More on transpersonal aspects of our unconscious and collective consciousness in Chapter 6 and 7.

[3] This link of our unconscious with our higher Self, collective consciousness, and the All is mentioned in passing here, as it relates to some of the major functions of the unconscious mind. Again, see further discussions in Chapter 6.

Pain as a Wakeup Call from the Unconscious

There is no coming to consciousness without pain.

—Carl Jung

The longer we use WHEE, the more we come to appreciate that our pain and distress are messages from our unconscious, inviting us to attend to some aspects of our lives that we have overlooked or neglected. These calls for attention from our inner being may include lessons at any or all of the wholistic levels of body, emotions, mind, relationships, and spirit.

Van was overweight and had high blood pressure and severe headaches. His headaches were related to his hypertension, as they disappeared when he took blood pressure medications. Talking with his headaches, Van came to accept that his deeper self was yelling at him through the headaches to do something about his weight and his blood pressure. The deeper lessons that followed involved issues of low self-esteem and loneliness that Van was covering up with comfort eating.

* * *

Holly had suffered for eight years from premenstrual pains of such severity that she was laid up in bed for one or two days each month. Medical workups revealed no cause for these pains, and several gynecological procedures failed to relieve them. Various hormones and pain pills also proved unhelpful as well as causing multiple annoying and unpleasant side effects.

Dialoguing with the pain uncovered a whole complex of lingering guilts and old, buried fears over a therapeutic abortion Holly had had at age 19, in her first year at a college away from home. She still felt guilty for not having told her boyfriend and for not having gone to confession. At the time she also had been extremely anxious and fearful that her parents would find out and might refuse to continue paying for her education.

WHEE immediately relieved the pains to the point that Holly no longer needed time off prior to her periods. She was able to deal successfully with all of the issues around the abortion, mostly using WHEE on her own, with a minimum of therapist guidance.

When the pains resisted clearing below a SUDS of 2, we then explored further for other psychological issues, uncovering an incident of molestation by a janitor in her Catholic elementary school. Her SUDS went up to a 9. Clearing her distress over this memory brought about complete clearance of her premenstrual pains.

Pain is one of the principal ways in which the unconscious mind draws our attention to dis-ease that underlies many of our physical problems in life. Obesity, hypertension, and menstrual problems are only a few examples of psychological issues that contribute to or cause symptoms and illnesses. Western medicine tends to focus on physical symptoms and diagnoses diseases—all of which it addresses through physical interventions.

Many have gotten so used to popping pills to solve their problems that they don't think of possible psychological issues that might be present. They also prefer the easier route of letting someone else tell them what is wrong and prescribing a "fix" for it. In many cases, this apparently easier route turns out to be a very costly one. You may recall the most serious consequences of 100,000 people dying annually in the US from medications "properly" prescribed.

On deeper levels, because people's Inner Child programs warn them away from their buried hurts, they often persist in their default patterns of running away from whatever is uncomfortable. I dearly hope that, one day soon, more people will benefit from the awareness and knowledge of WHEE, in addition to modern medicine, in dealing with their problems.

6

Spiritual Dimensions of WHEE and Pain

There comes a time in the spiritual journey when you start making choices from a very different place....And if a choice lines up so that it supports truth, health, happiness, wisdom, and love, it's the right choice.

—Angeles Arrien

In my explorations I have come to define personal spirituality as "an awareness of ourselves as extending beyond our physical body."[1] Within this definition, spiritual aspects of ourselves include: biological energies that surround and interpenetrate the body; intuitive awareness that transcends ordinary time and space; collective consciousness of humans; collective consciousness of nature; our own spirit and soul; communications with the spirits of people who have crossed from physical life into another dimension; nature spirits and angels; and God/the Divine/the Infinite Source/the eternal, omniscient, cosmic consciousness. Any and all of these can boost the effects of WHEE.

Coming in the other direction, WHEE can open and deepen our spiritual awareness and our connections with our personal and collective spirituality. It is not only through the practice of affirmations or inviting energies and agencies outside ourselves to help us that we connect with our spirituality. The process of incremental addition of these elements in the practice of WHEE provides a way to check whether they make any difference to us in releasing negatives and installing positives, and to what degree they do so.

---

[1] For more details, see *Healing Research, Volume 3.*

As we engage with our spirituality, we also come to an inner knowing that it is very real and potent. I use the term, *gnowing* to indicate an inner knowing that carries with it its own sense of validity. As we develop our intuitive senses, with feedback from our inner and outer worlds to validate our perceptions, we come to know and trust this kind of awareness. It is like learning to trust our sense of balance with our eyes closed. At first, visual feedback is helpful so that we can orient ourselves in the spaces around us. Soon, however, we come to trust our kinesthetic sense of the positions of our body parts. The internal feedback loops of WHEE can be a major help in this same sort of feedback process as we learn to trust where we are with our personal spiritual awareness in the world.

Connecting with our personal spirituality, validating its realities in our lives, deepening this awareness, learning to trust it, and connecting with the All may be the most important work of our lives. This is one of the reasons that WHEE is so potent and effective. It helps us to grow along the dimension of our personal spirituality, which is a vital aspect of our lives.

> *While life and all its vagaries are interesting, it is the growth of the Soul that is the essence of our purpose for gracing the Earth.*

> —Joellen Koerner

Personal spirituality may be unfamiliar to many who are raised in Western cultures, which focus our lives on thinking, analyzing, and dissecting our experiences, primarily emphasizing the physical aspects of our being. I am not addressing spirituality here through religious practices, although these may also help us to connect with our personal spiritual awareness. I am inviting you to experience your *personal* connection with the All, your participation as a pixel on the big screen of the Infinite Source.

As a pixel, we may be consciously aware of only a limited part of the picture of All that Is. Yet we are connected through our unconscious with everything, everywhere, everywhen. We know this with the inner consciousness that I call *gnowing*—the direct, intuitive knowledge that often carries with it an inner, numinous sense of certainty about its validity. For some, this awareness seems to arise from the intuitive right brain; for others it is a knowing felt in the heart rather than in the head. To those who have experienced gnosis, it may feel even more real than physical reality, which, in comparison, is sometimes described as an illusion.

If you have not tasted the fruit of the cactus or a persimmon, then whatever words I use to describe their flavors will remain mere words — descriptions and analogies to other experiences that you and I have lived. So it is with personal spirituality. Until you have connected with your personal gnowing of your part in the improvisational mystery theater co-created by each of us in collaboration with the Infinite Source, you will only know *about* it. WHEE invites you to explore this dimension for yourself in little paces, savoring your experience at every step. Using yourself as the instrument for exploration, you will become aware of, appreciate, and *know* that your gnowing is a real and potent part of your life.

The Hebrew word *ruach* means both *"wind" and "spirit."* Far from conincidental, this double meaning provides insight into the nature of personal spirituality: You cannot see the wind, but you can perceive its effects in the world as it rustles leaves, caresses or pushes strongly against your body, ripples sand dunes, and blows the clouds across the sky. So it is, too, with your awareness of the Infinite Source. You can know it by its effects upon your consciousness — whispering to you through intuition about your life and relationships; shouting at you with symptoms of pain and serious anxieties about lighter messages you may have not heard or ignored; and stopping you in your tracks with injuries or serious illnesses. All of these messages are calls to awaken and clear the blocks to our participation in the collective flow of energies and consciousness.

In each of the steps detailed below, you will be able to use the WHEE process to sense the effects of your personal spirituality on your SUDS and your SUSS. This will provide a measure for the power of the Infinite Source in your life. As with any other exploration with WHEE, it is helpful to do a few rounds on a difficult issue that goes down slowly in order to get a baseline sense of how fast your affirmation is working. Then, on the next round of WHEE, introduce a spiritual focus that appeals to you. Note both the intensity of the shift in SUDS and any qualitative differences in your responses. In this way, your diminishing pain or other issues will give you feedback on the power of spirituality in your life, when compared to when you did the WHEE initially on the same issue but without the spiritual component.

Biological Energies that Surround and Interpenetrate the Body

It is possible that there exist human emanations which are still un-known to us. Do you remember how electrical currents and "unseen waves" were laughed at? The knowledge about man is still in its infancy.

— Albert Einstein

Biological energies, or *bioenergies*, can be accessed within ourselves and may be offered by others to enhance our health in general and our pain management in particular. Healers and people who see or sense energies with their hands report that they perceive an energy field that surrounds and interpenetrates the body. Outside the body, the field is seen to have a series of layers that relate to various functions of the person: physical, emotional, mental, relational, and spiritual.

Disorders in the physical body, in psychological states, and in connections with other people and with one's spiritual self are reflected in alterations of the energy fields. For instance, physical trauma from a car accident may be associated with intense emotions. Pain may persist well beyond the time the tissues heal. Only when associated emotions and bioenergies are released will the pain abate. Elmer Green, one of the originators of biofeedback, called such trauma residues energy cysts. These can be released through interventions that address:

- the body (e.g. through self-healing such as biofeedback, or massage by a therapist)
- the emotions and mind (e.g. through bodymind psychotherapies, emotional releases, and systematic desensitization)
- the bioenergy field (e.g. through chakra healing, spiritual healing, craniosacral therapy, acupuncture, and its derivatives)
- WHEE is particularly effective because it is a wholistic approach and addresses all of these levels.

Abnormalities of biofields are often accompanied by pain. Healers may relieve pains by sensing blocks, excess flows, or sluggish flows of bioenergies, then correct these through interactions of their biofields with those of the healee. Research in Spiritual healing—as in Therapeutic Touch, Healing Touch, prayer, and similar methods—has been shown to relieve pains from surgery, arthritis, tension headaches, and various chronic, intractable conditions.[2]

---

[2] Current findings on this topic are reviewed in *Healing Research, Volume 1.*

Biofields can also be influenced and altered through our own intentions. One way is by enhancing WHEE through various self-healing biofields interventions. Several energetic points on the body correspond with different aspects of our physical, emotional, and mental experience. One of these is the releasing spot mentioned earlier—below the midpoint of the collarbone—where a massage often helps to release resistances. This is a potent acupressure point known for releasing negativity. Additionally, seven major charkas (bioenergy centers) along the midline of the body are associated with states of health and illness of nearby organs.

The *heart chakra* can be activated to enhance the effects of WHEE. While alternating tapping on each side of your body (e.g. with the index and middle finger of one hand touching the eyebrows across the bridge of your nose; tapping your feet on the floor; or tightening the toes on your right and left foot), you can enhance the effects of tapping by holding your other hand over your heart chakra. Explore how this influences your use of WHEE. Many have found this to be particularly potentiating in their explorations and easing of pains.

> **Exercise:** Do several rounds of WHEE on a challenging issue with a high SUDS. Use your eyebrow points or feet for the right-left tapping, so that one of your hands remains free. Then, hold a free hand over your heart chakra and repeat the same process, noting whether this enhances the rate of release of your SUDS or enhancement of your SUSS.

Earth Energies Can Strengthen Effects of WHEE

The Earth to us is an intelligent living being. It has a natural intelligence in itself, and it is able to talk to us, to communicate with us, to guide us in what to do—if we pray and open up to it and come into harmony with it.

—Sun Bear

Mother Earth/Gaia supports all life on this planet. We can tap into Earth energies by consciously connecting with them. While doing WHEE, we can invite Earth energies to rise through our feet, filling every aspect of our being. Many people report that this markedly potentiates the effects of WHEE. Check it out for yourself.

As many people confirm this works for them, we can begin to sense that our consciousness can activate helpful energies from outside ourselves. Earth energies can enhance your pain relief with WHEE.

Negative energies in the environment may be stressful. For example, when I rode the underground in London after work, the negative energies of tired, rushed, and otherwise unhappy people used to drain my system. Just as we can invite positive outside energies to help us, however, we can consciously block negative energies from draining or hurting us. A common way to do this is through imagery. Prior to going into a place of known negative energies, picture to yourself that there is an energy shield (like in Star Trek) surrounding your body and only allowing energies that are for your highest good to enter your energy field. This imagery served me well to block the influence of tired, negative energies on the London Underground!

Spiritual affirmations can also enhance WHEE. For instance, after saying, "I love and accept myself wholly and completely" you may add, "and God/the Divine/the Infinite Source loves and accepts me, wholly, completely, and unconditionally." Again, as with any other new element you choose to add to your WHEE procedure, use incremental explorations and tweak the words you use to confirm how helpful these are for you, checking how rapidly your SUDS is shifting.

Intuitive Awareness Validates Our Spiritual Awareness

Intuition comes as a certain feeling or a still voice.... If you use your intuition, you will know the very purpose for which you exist in this world; and when you find that, you find happiness.

— Paramahansa Yogananda

We connect with our inner, intuitive awareness in using the SUDS and SUSS assessments, muscle testing, and surrogate healing. When we find how effective our intuitive awareness is in guiding our inner processes, we grow to trust it.

With time, we come to have a sense of the validity of spiritual awareness. I find that there is a distinct quality of engagement with transcendent realities. I sense this in my personal use of intuition in psychotherapy and of offering and receiving spiritual healing. It resembles the sensory awareness of perceiving distinctive odors that identify particular experiences, such as the smell of wet, cut grass that accompanies the fresh mowing of a lawn or the smell of fearfulness in a tense, traumatic situation. There are times when this transcendent smell-like sense is strong and unmistakable, and other times when it may be weak to the point that it is difficult to be certain whether it is actually there.

The same is true of spirituality in dreams. Some dreams are accompanied by extra-sharp sensations, such as unusually vivid colors, colors that do not exist in the ordinary world, heavenly music (sometimes called *music of the spheres*), or the presence of spirit entities who bring us helpful and inspirational

Working on WHEE in a group is helpful in this regard. When several people work together, a group energy develops that facilitates opening into spiritual awareness, especially if all in the group are committed to this endeavor.

Psychokinesis and Healing

Mind shapes matter and body, so state your intentions and wishes clearly.

—Daniel J. Benor

Not only are we intimately interconnected with the world around us through ESP, but we also are able to influence the world around us without physical interventions through intent, meditation, and prayer. In popular terminology this is called *mind over matter*, and in parapsychology is labeled *psychokinesis* (PK).

Research on PK has produced impressive collections of formal research studies confirming that mental intent can literally influence the roll of dice, with subjects rolling randomly chosen faces of balanced dice far more often than chance would predict.[3] Similarly, the outputs of random number generators (RNGs) can be influenced through intent. RNGs produce equal numbers of zeros and ones when left to run on their own. However, if a person sits in front of the RNG and wills it to produce more ones or zeros, it deviates significantly from random output.[4] While these effects are only modest in any one trial, the

---

[3] Radin and Ferrari, 1991.
[4] Radin, 1997; Radin and Nelson, internet reference.

combined results from rigorous studies are a billion to one against the effects on dice being caused by chance, and a trillion to one in the studies on RNGs.

Put in everyday language, the research on mind over matter is highly convincing and very, very, very unlikely to have been caused by chance. One of the more fascinating discoveries is that, just as believers do, skeptics and disbelievers in PK produce significant results too—but their results are opposite those requested of them to produce.[5]

An impressive body of research also confirms that spiritual healing can produce significant effects on living organisms. In my annotated review of 191 scientific studies of healing[6] I found that when the 52 more rigorous reports were considered, 74 percent demonstrated significant effects of healing in humans, animals, plants, bacteria, yeasts, cells in laboratory culture, and enzymes.

Having studied spiritual healing for over 25 years, I am impressed that most people have some measure of this ability. A mother kissing away a child's hurt is giving healing; a compassionate word or touch carries healing; and the intent to help with WHEE can activate healing for ourselves and others.

Most interesting, but as yet unexplained, are the confirmed abilities of healers to send healing from any distance. This can be a part of WHEE, as in the next section below.[7] You might wish to do a simple experiment to explore your healing abilities:

Experiment: Fill three planting pots of equal size with equal amounts of potting soil from the same source. Number each one clearly with a label or marker. Sort out corn seeds of equal size from the same seed packet. Place an equal number of seeds in the soil of each container, being careful to position each seed with its pointy end down and flat end up, and to bury each to the same depth. Water each container with the same amount of water every one to three days, depending upon how fast they dry—being certain not to let the containers dry completely. See that each container gets an equal amount of light.

---

[5] Lawrence.

[6] Benor, 2001(a), 2001(b).

[7] See details on spiritual healing in *Healing Research, Volume 1, Scientific Validation of a Healing Revolution*.

If you have someone else to help you, let them handle the seeds, pots, and watering while you send your healing from a distance to one of the pots. *Do not disclose the number of the chosen pot to the plant-tender.*

Think positive, loving thoughts or project the wish to heal the first container. Ignore the second. Think angry or negative thoughts about the third. (Some prefer to omit the third.) If your healing ability with plants is strong, you should see a noticeable difference between the speed at which seeds germinate and the amount of growth at the end of two weeks. Results may vary when you give healing at different times of day, and under different phases of the moon.

Spiritual healing is an outstanding intervention that often alleviates distressing symptoms such as pain, stress, and distress. It is safe, with no known harmful effects. My one caution in using healing is that is has the potential for disempowering some people who seek external solutions for their problems. Many healers and healees work in a manner similar to the medical model, in which the therapist is expected to "fix" the "patient." WHEE has the advantage of empowering you to help yourself rather than relying on someone else to do this for you. When spiritual healing is used as a booster to WHEE or other treatments that require a therapist (such as massage, acupuncture, homeopathy, and so on), I feel that it is making a contribution that is not as likely to be disempowering.

People often ask, "How can you explain spiritual healing?" The honest answer is, we don't yet know. Healing appears to act through bioenergies and intention. Distant healings appears to act through the collective consciousness of our planet, and more clearly includes the participation of the Infinite Source.[8]

Proxy/Surrogate Healing

Wishes and prayers are potent interventions, not to be taken lightly.

—Daniel J. Benor

Proxy healing can allow you to help others indirectly with your practice of WHEE. It is important, however, to have the other person's

---

[8] More on this in *Healing Research, Volumes 1 and 3.*

permission—or, if they are not competent to give their consent themselves, to get the consent of their guardian—before you offer Proxy WHEE. Here are the steps for this way of helping:

1. Connect with the other person through intent. You can do this simply by saying, "I am [*insert name*]."

2. Use WHEE on yourself, as though you were actually the other person using WHEE on her- or himself. If they have pain, you might say, "Even though I have this pain [*describing it as specifically as you would for yourself, to the best of your knowledge of the other person's experience*], I love and accept myself," and so on. The other person will have the benefits of the WHEE process.

3. At the end of your WHEE surrogate series, disconnect yourself from the other person by affirming, "I am no longer [*insert the other person's name*], I am [*insert your own name*]."

Here are some examples of how WHEE can be used in proxy healing:

> Jimmie was two years old. He had suffered second-degree burns when he scalded his face, chest, and belly by pulling down a pot of boiling water from the stove when his mother left the kitchen to answer the phone. He was terrified of dressing changes because of the pain he had experienced with his first dressing change in the hospital. I instructed his mother in using proxy WHEE, and she was able to calm his fears within minutes.

* * *

> Gilda's tabby cat, Zebra, was aging and clearly slowing down but still able to get around and enjoy her feline routines of watching birds wistfully from the window and making her way up to the dining room table via a chair when it remained pulled out after a meal. When Zebra started dripping urine between her normal visits to the litter box, Gilda became distressed. Fortunately, she was able to cure this with proxy WHEE, with the focusing statement, "Even though I'm wetting the floor...."

How WHEE helps with symptoms such as an aging cat's weak control over her bladder sphincter is beyond my explanation. However, it is not uncommon for WHEE and other Energy Psychology methods to produce such effects.[9]

The ethics of offering WHEE in this way are an issue deserving some thought. While some people feel comfortable sending healing wishes or prayers to anyone, my feeling is that this ought to be done only with permission. We would not push a pill into someone's mouth because we thought it might help them. Similarly, we ought not lay a healing wish on someone when this might influence them in ways that are not of their choosing.

Past-life Memories Can Enhance the Effects of WHEE

A bodily disease may be but a symptom of some ailment in the spiritual past.

—Nathaniel Hawthorne

While Western society has lost much of its awareness of memories from past lives that can influence present life issues, Eastern traditions accept reincarnation as a part of the path of human existence. Various prominent Westerners have written about these connections, including: Louisa May Alcott, Elizabeth Barrett Browning, Charles Dickens, Arthur Conan Doyle, George Elliot, Ralph Waldo Emerson, Victor Hugo, David Hume, William James, Henry Wadsworth Longfellow, Edgar Allen Poe, Alfred Lord Tennyson, Henry David Thoreau, Leo Tolstoy, Voltaire, Walt Whitman, and John Greenleaf Whittier, among others. Notable figures from the more distant past to have touched upon the subject include Cicero, Plato, and Pythagoras.

I was surprised and intrigued to discover that a variety of research approaches have confirmed past-life memories.[10] I present only a few of these fascinating details here.

Spontaneous reincarnation memories were investigated by Ian Stevenson, a psychiatrist at the University of Virginia. Stevenson pioneered explorations of such cases from India, Lebanon, Sri Lanka, and other cultures around the world. He meticulously collected first-hand

---

[9] Surrogate healing is also commonly offered through spiritual healing, discussed in *Healing Research, Volume 1.*

[10] These studies are reviewed in detail in my book *Healing Research, Volume 3: Personal Spirituality.*

accounts of witnesses who corroborated the telling and/or demonstrating of such memories. He found numerous cases in which multiple witnesses verified the reported events.[11] Particularly impressive are the cases of children who recall a previous life, in societies where there is little access to the media and little mobility.

Hypnotic regressions to previous lives have been reported for decades. Psychotherapists may regress people to past lives in order to help them resolve emotional and relationship problems. Typically, people will present themselves to their therapist with a persistent pain, phobia, anxiety, or interpersonal conflict that has not responded to conventional counseling approaches. The therapist helps them awaken relevant experiences that are apparently lingering in their unconscious mind from previous lifetimes. People will frequently experience intense emotional releases as they recall traumatic past-life experiences, such as their own death or the death of a dear one. Bringing out the related memories and feelings often frees people of their presenting problems.

> Sonya suffered from pains around her left shoulder blade for years. These had begun shortly after her breakup with her boyfriend, who abandoned her for another woman. In a past-life regression, Sonya recalled being betrayed and stabbed in the back in a political conflict in France in the seventeenth century. In releasing her feelings of betrayal from the earlier life experiences, she was able also to release those same feelings from her rejection by her boyfriend. Her back pain was gone at the end of the session.

Past-life memories can be elicited in many cases just by inviting people to look for them. Using current issues as cues, people will go to the filing cabinet drawer and pull out the relevant earlier life memories.

Psychics and mediums often identify past-life events that are relevant to current-life issues. Denys Kelsey, a psychiatrist, was a noted past-life therapist who was married to the late Joan Grant, a gifted psychic. They worked as a team. When Kelsey had patients whose problems were not resolved in psychoanalytic therapy, he called in his wife. She psychically read their past lives for traumatic events that seemed relevant to their current-life conflicts. They found that numerous problems

---

[11] Stevenson, 1987.

and symptoms that were unresponsive to conventional psychotherapy were rapidly resolved in this way.[12]

Research on past-life hypnotic regressions has produced some fascinating results. Helen Wambach gathered two large groups of past-life memories under group hypnosis in Southern California. One series had 850 cases; the other had 350. Wambach sorted them first by century and within each century distributed them geographically. In each geographic area she sifted the cases into their apparent socio-economic groups. These sortings produced percentages of upper, middle, and lower classes that closely parallel what is known of population distributions in the respective historical periods. Gender distribution in past lives was split 50 percent male/female in both groups, although the real-life distribution in her first series was 78 percent female. Wambach also studied clothing, food, and other items mentioned in past-life recall. There were cases in which verified types of historical items were mentioned that the subjects claimed they had had no conscious knowledge of prior to the hypnotic regressions. There were very few cases of objects misplaced in time.[13]

Wambach's findings contradict skeptics' views that people are just making up these memories. If that were the case, I would expect typical Southern Californians who are out for a reincarnation experience to imagine they were of the same gender as in their current life, to be of at least middle-class in dress, and to be geographically distributed with a skew to Europe and the Americas, perhaps with a generous sprinkling of lives in the land of the Bible. None of these predictions was supported.

Numerous explorers in these realms have come to the conclusion that reincarnation appears to be the process of spirits and souls taking the equivalent of elective courses in the material world, with a major in spiritual development. Explorations through reincarnation and near-death studies, along with evidence from channeled reports and possession provide glimpses of what it is like to be alive in spirit between earthly lives.

WHEE can be helpful in releasing feelings from past-life memories, just as it helps with current-life memories. The release of such buried

---

[12] Kelsey and Grant, 1967.
[13] Wambach, 1979.

traumatic emotions may release pains and other symptoms in our current lives, just as the release of buried memories and feelings from our current life may relieve such symptoms.

I started out a horrible skeptic about intuitive and spiritual matters, not having been inspired by my family or religion to connect with these, and having been indoctrinated by my education and training in psychology, medicine, psychiatry, and research in materialistic views and theories about the world. Over the years, as I moved from learning about spiritual healing to developing my own healing gifts and integrating them with psychotherapy, my spiritual awareness deepened.

While I believed in reincarnation, I had not had any direct past-life memories myself until one day my unconscious mind opened my awareness through my body. I was out bicycling and fell as the bike was climbing up over the curb from the road. Luckily, I landed on grass, taking most of the impact on the outside of my left upper thigh, almost at the hip. I thought little of the fall, and without any difficulties or discomfort rode about three or four miles back home.

Over the next few days, my left thigh and hip area started aching. I thought this was not unusual, as I had experienced such injuries in the past with a similar cause. However, when the pains worsened rather than abating after several more days, and when the pain shifted slightly from one location to another, it became clear to me that something energetic was happening.

With the help of a gifted medical intuitive, I was encouraged to ask my unconscious mind to reveal any memories or images that might be associated with this pain. To my great surprise, I saw myself as a Native American or First Nation man in my late twenties or early thirties, trekking with others in a clan up a mountain snowscape. I had injured my left thigh and was finding it increasingly difficult to keep up with the others.

The leader of the clan called a halt and we discussed the situation. The clan had to move forward to its next camp by nightfall. This was not a choice but a necessity for survival in the sub-freezing weather. There were no pack animals or other resources to carry me. There was no alternative but for me to accept that I would either follow as best I could or make my peace with the Creator and give up my life on that cold mountainside.

I had no hard feelings towards the clan. This was the way of our life in that place and time. Individuals had to be sacrificed if their conditions threatened the survival of the whole group. So we said our farewells and I settled into the hollow of a tree to rest and see if I could muster the strength to climb any further. The pain was only worse after resting, and I realized that my end was near.

While I was not angry with the clan, I was angry with the Creator. I had married into this clan only a couple of years earlier. My wife and child died in childbirth, and I had not bonded nearly as strongly with the rest of the clan as I had with my wife. As I settled in to my tree hollow to die of the cold, which was not that terrible a death as deaths in those days and circumstances could be, I felt I had been abandoned by the Creator.

It took me a number of weeks of inner work to sort through my feelings from this past-life memory that resonated strongly with experiences of abandonment in my current life, including the distant relationships I had with my parents, as well as several partnered relationships that ended against my wishes.

WHEE was extremely helpful to me both in clearing the feelings from the past-life memory and peeling deeper layers of the onion of feelings from these and other, related issues in my current life that I had worked on earlier.

My own experience is supported by thousands of reports from many other therapists. Releases of traumas from past-life memories provides release of symptoms in one's current life that are identical to the releases of symptoms experienced when WHEE reduces the SUDS of traumatic memories and feelings that were experienced in current lives.

Past-life memories raise fascinating questions. The first, in our society, is: *Are these memories real?* The story of my wintry death on the mountain could be pure fantasy, created by my mind out of my life circumstances. In psychological lingo this is termed a *screen memory*—a false memory that creates an explanatory myth, which is helpful in sorting out or explaining away uncomfortable feelings from experiences in one's current life. Alternatively, it could have been a simple fantasy that I created, stimulated by the intuitive's suggestion.

I have no way to disprove these theories. I can only say that this memory helped me do a major inner housecleaning job around feelings of rejection.

As to general questions about the reality of reincarnation memories, there is a wealth of evidence, reviewed briefly above, suggesting that these are real memories. What is even more impressive to me is that these studies have been replicated with children and adults by researchers in the US, England, France, Germany, Australia, South America, Russia, and many other places around the world. The evidence is consistent and coherent.

As relevant to WHEE, traumatic residues from reincarnation memories (be they real or fantasized) can be released just as easily as current-life residues. Again, WHEE may be much faster than many other past-life therapy methods.

Death Has a Bad Reputation

Pain and death are part of life. To reject them is to reject life itself.

—Havelock Ellis

The belief that death is the end of existence has produced enormous suffering in Western culture. People fear death, and anything related to death and dying becomes a prime item for avoidance and burying outside of conscious awareness. These fears contribute to anxieties around serious illnesses, which make people uptight and worsen their experiences of pains that may be a part of such illnesses.

Friends and relatives may likewise be afraid of death—of the approaching end of physical life of the person who is ill and of their own. So they will often tiptoe around the fact that the ill person is moving toward their final breaths in this lifetime, afraid of upsetting him or themselves. The ill person, sensing their discomfort, will likewise avoid this subject.

These fears prevent the wonderful clearings of unresolved issues that can unfold between family and friends as death approaches. Where fears of death are not present or can be overcome, we can work through feelings and memories that have lingered on the shelves and in the caves where we set them down out of discomfort in dealing with them. The weeks and days prior to a person's death can bring deep healings to the person who is dying and to everyone associated with him or her. Then, the pain of old, unspoken hurts, resentments, and angers can be cleared and we can each come to our own place of understanding, acceptance, and forgiveness.

WHEE can be of enormous help in dealing with unresolved feelings and memories at such times. This is not an avoidance of feeling or issues, but a deep clearing of whatever is discomforting or hurting.

> *Center of all centers, core of cores,*
> *almond self-enclosed and growing sweet-*
> *all this universe, to the furthest stars*
> *and beyond them is your flesh, your fruit.*
>
> *Now you feel how nothing clings to you;*
> *Your vast shell reaches into endless space,*
> *And there the rich, thick fluids rise and flow.*
> *Illuminated in your infinite peace.*
>
> *A billion stars go spinning through the night,*
> *blazing high above your head.*
> *But in you is the presence that*
> *will be, when all the stars are dead.*

—Rainer Maria Rilke

The issue of possible suicide may arise in discussions of death, particularly where severe and unrelenting pains are present. Practical issues of discussing suicide and providing support for dealing with pain have already been considered at the end of Chapter 2. In this chapter, we will consider the spiritual aspects of suicide.

Where religious or personal beliefs of the person in pain do not condemn suicide, questions arise about the consequences of such a choice and action within a framework of personal spirituality. I have been exploring spiritual beliefs and practices for thirty years, including discussions with many people and omnivorous reading. What I have learned from those who have had near-death experiences—which I consider to be the closest we can come to first-hand knowledge and opinions about death—has led me to believe that suicide is not condemned, but is definitely discouraged in the realms to which we transition after physical death. We are given challenges in our lives that are lessons for our souls. These challenges are carefully chosen prior to our birth by our higher selves, in consultation with guides in spirit and higher realms. It is said that we are not given challenges that are greater than our abilities to handle them. If we elect to end our life so that we will not suffer pains, we may be invited to "repeat the course" we opted out of in this lifetime. This is not a spiritual failure or a sin. It is simply a require-ment that has somehow been agreed for the progress and development of our soul. If we do not learn the lessons in one lifetime, we are then given other chances to learn them.

Within a religious or cultural framework that holds suicide as a sin, it may be very challenging and difficult for family members of a person who contemplates suicide to deal with this issue. The help of a counselor who can support the person in pain can be enormously helpful. My own approach is never to judge anyone who is involved, but to be present to facilitate discussions and the sharing of feelings so all present know that they have been heard.

At the opposite end of the spectrum is the person who is in pain but lingers long beyond the time predicted by medical authorities for their survival. This is a lesson to all in the wholistic nature of life. While the physical body may be ravaged by disease, the mind and spirit may cling to life. When this happens, it very often is due to the wish of the ill person to survive for particular reasons. Research shows that far more people die after a major holiday such as Easter or Passover than before the celebration. In other cases, people hold on because of their wishes to complete a task or obligation.

Another force for lingering in pre-death may be the wishes of family members to hold onto the person, or fears surrounding their impending death. When family members come to a point of acceptance, the dying person may be freed to depart.

Jewish tradition holds that prayer can stave off death. An example is the story of Rabbi Yehuda Hanassi, who lay unconscious on his deathbed, barely clinging to life. His disciples were loath to see him leave this earth and kept a constant prayer vigil to prevent his spirit from departing. His wife, seeing him in distress, prayed that his soul might depart but as his disciples continued to pray for his soul to remain, her prayer was not answered. She then took a large jug and sent it crashing to the floor. This momentarily silenced their prayers and the Rabbi's soul departed.

Death is a natural part of life. Where we are fearful of dealing with our feelings about death, tensions and pains are generated. WHEE can be helpful in dealing with these, again converting worries into concerns that are more manageable.

Clearing Unresolved Issues with Spirits

Anger cannot occur unless you believe that you have been attacked, that your attack is justified in return, and that you are in no way responsible for it. Given these three wholly irrational premises, the equally irrational conclusion that a brother is worthy of attack rather than of love must follow. What can be expected from insane premises except an insane conclusion? The way to undo an insane conclusion is to consider the sanity of the premises on which it rests. You cannot be attacked, attack has no justification, and you are responsible for what you believe.

—*A Course in Miracles*

It is possible to work through unresolved conflicts with people from our current and past lives who are now in spirit existence. With the help of WHEE we can dialogue with them and release the feelings that arise within us. We can use proxy healing to help them release their unresolved feelings. These releases, as with the clearing of past life memories, may have profound healing effects.

When invited to do so, many people can very quickly connect with an inner awareness of relatives and friends on the other side of the veil. This is similar to connecting with past-life awareness. If this does not work for you, it is possible to consult an intuitive counselor who can facilitate such communications. It is then possible to use WHEE to reduce residual tensions, angers, hurts, and other feelings or issues that were unresolved when they were still present in the flesh.

Peter's father had been physically and emotionally abusive in his childhood. Peter had spent years in therapy to overcome his post-traumatic stress disorder, which included multiple fears around loud and aggressive people, low self-esteem, inability to assert himself both personally and professionally, and various self-defeating behaviors. Since his father remained abusive, Peter cut off his relationship with him, moving to a distant city.

Toward the end of his life, his father mellowed—according to reports that Peter heard from his brother and sisters. Peter still refused to have anything to do with him, even to the point of not attending his father's funeral.

Years after his father's death, through working in counseling on issues with his own children, Peter came to a place of forgiveness for his father. He realized that his father had had an enormously difficult childhood himself, having been abandoned by his abusive, alcoholic parents and having suffered further abuse in various foster homes through most of his growing-up years.

Peter was intrigued, though skeptical, about using WHEE to resolve his residual distress with his father. He figured he had nothing to lose, however, in exploring this possibility. To his surprise, he was able to open to awareness of his father's presence by entering a quiet, meditative state. He found his father much mellower than he had ever experienced in their relationship before. He was very disappointed, however, when his father denied having been as abusive as Peter recalled he had been. Peter was looking for his father to acknowledge having hurt Peter and to ask for forgiveness.

Peter asked his father if it would be okay to help him release any leftover feelings he might have from his difficult childhood. Peter explained that he had had great success with WHEE in releasing his own challenging issues. Though skeptical, his father agreed.

Peter held his awareness of his father's presence and did proxy healing on angers, resentments, and hurts that his father reported he still carried. Both were surprised at how quickly these cleared. (Spirits, like children in earth-plane existence, often release issues rapidly with WHEE.) There was a distinct further softening in his father's responses to Peter. At the end of a second WHEE session, his father was able to ask forgiveness of Peter for any hurts he had caused, although still denying any recall of these. This made an enormous difference to Peter, who came away feeling greatly relieved of his burden of resentments toward his father.

With all such communications it is, of course, prudent to hold the awareness that our expectations, doubts, anxieties, or fears may impede or distort these dialogues across dimensions of space, time, and consciousness. While it is impossible to validate them in the same ways we validate communications in the flesh, the shifts in our inner states and the decreases in SUDS levels can confirm our successes through resolving our issues.

There is also a caution in choosing a spiritual counselor who is ethical and reliable. Some have been known to fabricate such communications for monetary gain, preying upon the vulnerabilities of the bereaved. Notable caution or alarm signals include the insistence on frequent sessions (rather than giving you the choice) and demands for excessively high fees.

Spiritual Bypass and Spiritual Inflation

You need to be a somebody before you can become a nobody.

—Brant Cortright

Explorations in spiritual realms are not without their complications. Some people become entranced with the thrills of spiritual explorations and pursue these to the exclusion of doing their personal inner work of clearing psychological issues. I call this a *spiritual bypass*.

I have seen spiritual bypasses often in people who are following paths of religious teachings and practices. Here, there may be the beliefs that abiding by religious commandments and going for absolution of sins is all that is needed to enter the gates of heaven. In my own tradition of birth in Judaism, one must ask forgiveness of one's fellow man before asking God for forgiveness on Yom Kippur, the annual fasting day of repentance. Even where practiced, this leaves 364 other days in the year when many ignore this requirement.

I have also seen spiritual bypasses in people pursing paths of personal spirituality. For instance, there may be an over-investment in spiritual rituals and practices, and in doing community work, with various degrees of neglect for self-exploration to clear psychological and relational issues. This may help to explain some of the glaring faults in prominent spiritual teachers.

On the other side of this issue, there are the dangers of ego infla-
tions through self-congratulation over spiritual achievements or asso-
ciations with particular spiritual teachers and schools.

> The two greatest challenges faced today by many spiritual seekers are
> arguably the danger of spiritual narcissism and the failure to integrate
> spiritual experiences into their everyday life. An inadequate assimila-
> tion of spiritual energies often leads to subtle forms of self-absorption
> and inflation, as well as to an increased, and often insatiable, thirst for
> spiritual experiences.
>
> —Jorge Ferrer

These issues are broader than space allows for full consideration
here. Instead, I offer a simple word of caution to those who might be
drawn toward over-investment in spiritual pursuits through the practice of WHEE.

Collective Consciousness

> Strength of heart comes from knowing that the pain that we each
> must bear is part of the greater pain shared by all that lives. It is not
> just "our" pain but "the" pain, and realizing this awakens our universal
> compassion.
>
> —Jack Kornfield

Our participation in collective consciousness can be considered
from several directions: 1. Our personal contributions to this super-con-
sciousness; and 2. The part we play in manifesting into the world that
which the collective consciousness wants to experience.

Our personal contributions to collective consciousness are often
outside our conscious awareness. It may take quite a bit of study, both
through personal experiences and more formal learning through books,
lectures, and workshops, to become aware of these levels of realities.

As a wholistic therapist (including spiritual awareness and healing
in psychotherapy, and addressing all levels of my own and of my clients' beingness), I'm keenly aware that we tend to manifest in the outer
world that which we need to learn in the inner world. I have marveled
at the outrageous synchronicities and manifestations in my life and
those of my clients that have reflected our inner conflicts, anxieties,

fears and other negativities as well as our positive feelings, wishes, healing awareness, and love.

Synchronicities are coincidences that have special meaning for the participants. I have had books that I sought to find, unsuccessfully, for days or weeks and months, appear without any effort on my part. I have met people I know from distant places in equally distant places for them, for no apparent reason. I have had songs and melodies playing on my radio that startlingly complemented or counterpointed events unfolding in my life and relationships at those very moments...to mention only a few common synchronicities.

Manifestations are appearances of material objects or of events that a person has asked for, and that have appeared through such unusual coincidences that they appear synchronistic. The books that appeared when I was seeking them would be an example of this.

Therapeutic encounters offer a wealth of opportunities for synchronicities. Here is an example from my clinical experience: It is very common to have clients show up who are seeking help with problems that closely parallel my own issues that I am at that time focused on clearing. At other times, clients may raise issues that resonate deeply in me and stir me to work on them. Many times I have been mildly stirred by a client's issues but did not feel moved to work on them myself. Within a very short time, a second and even a third client will show up with very similar problems—demanding my attention through persistence rather than intensity of presentations.

I recall clearly having a series of three such clients who stirred me to work on several layers of forgiveness of my mother for being very self-centered and unable to even recognize my emotional needs much less to respond to them in nurturing or healing ways. I found the first two clients remarkable in their spontaneously having arrived at states of forgiveness toward seriously abusive parents. The third client was struggling with angers and resentments, and through WHEE was able to reach a place of forgiveness very quickly. This was a great surprise to him, as he had carried these resentments for more than four decades.

I have a rule of threes: if something happens three times in short succession, I welcome it as a message that the universe is sending my way, calling my attention to explore whatever might be contained in the three similar incidents. Responding to the three messages from the collective consciousness about forgiveness, I delved inside and found further layers of forgiveness of my own that were ripe and waiting for me to work on and release: anger at my boss who had just made changes that affected my work, without consulting me; and hurt and anger towards my wife, who had done the same. I would not have done this work without the three prompts.

To explain these synchronicities stretches the limits of conventional understanding of the world. Many people dismiss them as pure coincidences. They believe that with the myriads of human interactions in our lives, there are bound to be some that strike us as unusual, and some that felicitously coincide with our needs and wishes or are so startling that they stir us to look at ourselves more closely.

I am convinced that consciousness is an organizing force in the universe. I believe the influence of consciousness extends beyond our physical selves, evidenced by the research on extrasensory perception and from the wealth of rigorous research demonstrating that intention and prayer can shape the healing of illnesses in humans and animals and the growth of plants, bacteria, and yeasts.

Our personal selves are interlinked with All that Is on every level of our being. When we don't process and clear our inner states at the level of our emotional, mental, and spiritual awareness, we manifest them into our bodies and into our relationships.[14] Coming from the opposite direction with WHEE, we may arrive at glimpses or deep reconnections with our spiritual path in life as we clear the inner and outer conflicts we have manifested into the world. This process provides direct personal awareness of the blocks and disconnections we set up earlier in our lives, distancing or separating us from our awareness of being one with the All. As we clear our defenses, we again experience the blessings and wonderful lessons we can manifest by being one with the flow of all creation.

Many examples of buried feelings that festered in the unconscious mind and then manifested in physical and relational problems have been presented in this book. I believe that this process occurs similarly within relationships of couples, families, institutions, and nations, through the

---

[14] See further discussion of my wholistic views of the interrelationships between body, emotions, mind, relationships, and spirit by clicking on round icons at the top of the websites www.ijhc.org or www.wholistichealingresearch.com.

same collective consciousness that brings about the individual reso-nations of outer with inner.

When we have hurts, angers and hatreds that are experienced col-lectively, these can fester into an outward focus of blaming "others" for our problems. This works through social mechanisms of interpersonal and media communications, as well as through psychic connections via the collective consciousness. These collective projections of our feel-ings can then lead us to attack those we designate as "others" in order to discharge some of our angers. Such lashing out, however, does not release the underlying, festering feelings of hurts. I hope that the per-sonal benefits and lessons of WHEE and related techniques will eventu-ally extend to cultural de-stressing and transformation of negativity on national and international levels.

Without such work to clear our angers, we tend to get into layers of vicious circles. Venting personal angers reduces our tensions. We feel better—in the sense of feeling less uptight or upset—for having discharged the tensions in our minds and bodies. The reduction in tension is experienced as a reward that strengthens our tendencies to repeat the angry behaviors. (This is like the unconscious rewards that got the teacher to move to the side of the classroom where the students were smiling.)

The social collective consciousness of our family, community, and nation—which is a limited sub-section of the vast, unconscious collec-tive consciousness discussed above—further reinforces angry behav-iors. When people around us are venting angers at "others" whom we feel justified in attacking, we feel validated in these behaviors of blam-ing and venting our angers upon those we designate as deserving such treatments. We repeat the behaviors and they become more strongly reinforced and entrenched.

Political leaders play upon these vicious circles by stirring anxieties and blaming someone outside our community, social class, race, or nation as the cause of our problems. This enables them to focus our angers and encourage us to vent them through war. Their true moti-vations, however, are often to profit through arms manufacturers, distract people from incompetencies of leadership that are the actual causes of the problems blamed on "others," and to enable leaders to enact laws giving them more power—all of which we would not otherwise agree to.

Beware the leader who bangs the drums of war in order to whip the citizenry into a patriotic fervor, for patriotism is indeed a double-edged sword. It both emboldens the blood, just as it narrows the mind....

And when the drums of war have reached a fever pitch and the blood boils with hate and the mind has closed, the leader will have no need in seizing the rights of the citizenry. Rather, the citizenry, infused with fear and blinded with patriotism, will offer up all of their rights unto the leader, and gladly so.

—Anonymous

These vicious circles get more vicious with time. One has only to look at the conflicts between Israelis and Arabs in the Middle East, Protestants and Catholics in Ireland, Hutus and the Tutsis in Rwanda, to mention a very few examples, to observe how the self-reinforcing behavior of letting angers out on inter-community and international levels can sadly perpetuate and worsen itself. Those who are attacked in anger feel justified in attacking back—whereupon the original attackers feel more justified in attacking again.

Stopping these vicious circles of anger begins on an individual level. We can learn to identify and release many of our own upsets through self-healing approaches such as WHEE. Then, we do not need to find outside targets to justify our venting angers. If enough of us do this, the world will not be such an explosively angry place.

On the positive side of the broader collective consciousness, we are all interconnected with every living and non-living aspect of our planet. In traditional cultures it is taken for granted that we are all part of our environment. We in Western cultures have only begun recently to reconnect in our awareness with *Gaia*, the collective consciousness that is our living planet, with everything on and in it. This is an important awareness for the healing of our planet—from our overpopulation, careless over-use of many resources, and pollution. WHEE helps us to reconnect with our spiritual awareness and can thus bring more healing to our planet.

In healing our planet, we also are healing ourselves. A substantial body of evidence shows that many illnesses are precipitated and/or worsened by the weakening of our immune systems due to environmental pollution. This brings us full circle in that the use of WHEE may contribute to raising spiritual awareness, which can lessen the toxins in our environment, which will lead to less cancer, arthritis, fibromyalgia, migraines, and other painful illnesses.

Our participation as brain cells in the mind of the collective consciousness may be more difficult to sense and appreciate than our personal contributions to these levels of awareness and experience. This sort of consciousness develops with our opening more deeply into spiritual awareness. Through meditation and in spontaneous awakenings — such as near death experiences — we may sense our participation in the Infinite Source. WHEE can help us to quiet our minds so that we may reach into these dimensions.[15]

Deeper Questions Raised by Pain

Pain nourishes courage. You can't be brave if you've only had wonderful things happen to you.

— Mary Tyler Moore

In addition to helping with the sensations of pain, WHEE can be helpful with the stresses and challenges of rearranging your life around your pain. Major experiences of pain, particularly when they are chronic, may stop us in our tracks — physically, energetically, emotionally, mentally, and socially. Pain can grab our complete attention, slow us down, and may even bring our life as we knew it to a halt. We may have to move slowly and carefully to avoid stirring up the pain and worsening it. We may have to plan carefully to avoid anything that increases our worries or tensions, and thereby increases our pain or decreases our tolerance for it. We may have to depend on others to help us with chores and work that we cannot manage without aggravating our pain. If the pain persists, then people we considered to be close may turn out to be fair weather friends. We may have to sort through shifting relationships, since not everyone will tolerate our pain, even when we don't consciously do anything to express our suffering, impose our pain experiences upon them, or make unusual demands.

---

[15] More on personal spiritual awareness in *Healing Research, Volume 3.*

In love's service only the wounded soldier can serve.

—Bernie Siegel, MD

It may be difficult to understand why friends and family find it difficult to be around us when we are in pain. There will, of course, be many individual answers to this question. In general, I observe that people who have not experienced severe pain or suffering, and have not been around others who are, simply do not understand what it is like for someone who is in pain. Some may feel they are failures for not being able to alleviate the pain; some may not know how to handle their own distress at seeing someone dear to them who is suffering; others may simply not want to be disturbed by having to deal with someone who is not in a positive space.

Severe and chronic pains, along with serious diseases that may cause them, also confront us with our mortality. We can no longer drive through life on automatic cruise control. We may be limited in our activities, which forces us to rearrange our lives and to accept that we may never again be able to enjoy some of the things we were able to do—to the same extent or at all. We may start to ask ourselves questions about the meaning of life and may address our mortality in deeper ways. This may also be a factor in making it difficult for others to deal with our pain, as the same feelings are raised for them. This may happen totally outside their conscious awareness. Their childhood programs of running away from what is painful may kick in, and they then avoid the person who is in pain in order not to suffer themselves.

Any and all of these issues may bring us to connect with our beliefs and questions about what happens after physical death. We may reconsider the religious teachings of our upbringing, either reconnecting with beliefs and practices that were or have been nurturing and sustaining, or distancing ourselves from these as we find new explanations and meanings for life that better fit our current situations, circumstances, and understandings.

All of these shifts and changes may be stressful and psychologically painful, in and of themselves. Again, WHEE can help with these issues, along with whatever else you find in your file drawers as you address the pain.

In addition to converting our anxieties, worries, and fears into more manageable concerns, WHEE can help us to connect more strongly with our personal spiritual awareness. As mentioned, earlier, repeating counteracting positives and replacement positives that include "[God/Christ/Mary/Buddha/Allah/my higher self] loves and accepts me, wholly, completely, and unconditionally" while tapping is a powerful way to do this.

The incremental addition of spiritual affirmation positives into a series of rounds of WHEE invites us to observe how this affects us. Many people can immediately sense a distinctly positive qualitative difference in the reductions of their SUDS and increases in their SUSS as they deliberately open to connect with their personal spiritual awareness.

Reducing and eliminating our anxieties, fears, pains, and limiting beliefs also removes blocks to connecting with our spirituality. I have seen many people come into a very quiet, meditative, spiritual space when they release their negative issues down to zero.

To round out this discussion on deeper aspects of the pain experience, let me share a few philosophical musings. I have always wondered whether we are doing the best thing by systematically working to reduce pains and eliminate them. Having shared all of the above, and having invested enormous efforts over many years in helping others to address their pains, and having worked diligently on my own pains, I am keenly aware of the wonderful lessons that pains have brought me and many others.

> You can hold back from the suffering of the world, you have permission to do so, and it is in accordance with your nature. But perhaps this very holding back is the one suffering you could have avoided.
>
> —Franz Kafka

Suffering deepens and heightens our awareness of our personal path. It pushes us to ask existential questions about why we are here in this world, about our relationships with other people and our life's mission. It is often a stimulus to creativity. It is certainly a profound teacher of compassion for others and a major motivator to help others who are suffering. I am reminded of the many people who have suffered emotional and physical pains, who came to feel that these were very positive, life-changing, and life-enhancing experiences. Numerous people with severe pains and serious illnesses have come to places of grace in which they are even thankful for having had the help of their pains in reshaping their lives. Here are but a few of the comments I have heard:

- "I never imagined I could ever say such a thing, but I am actually grateful I got this cancer. It stopped me in my tracks when I was living—in retrospect—an extremely busy but empty life. I have come to sense what life is really about. I am much more deeply happy now, even though I have this illness and have suffered all the horrible treatments you could imagine."

- "I tend to default to automatic pilot. I think most people do. I traveled through much of my life like when I drive a car and suddenly realize I wasn't really there for a bunch of miles. My pain keeps me very much awake and aware of my senses, my options, and my choices in life."

- "My pains and illness remind me that my hourglass of life is emptying. They help me stay on the edge of awareness where I choose, moment to moment, what is truly important and what I want to include in the time I have left on earth."

- "I think I have lived more—truly lived, with conscious awareness—in the few months of my pain and illness than in all the previous decades of my life."

The good thing about WHEE is that it is a delicate tool that allows us to address our issues selectively, at whatever level of suffering we would like to alleviate. Should you decide that your pain is in some measure a help in your life, you could use WHEE at the meta-level of decreasing your conflicts and expectations about eliminating your pain or about your distress, annoyance, or fears over having the pain. When we don't fret over our pains, they are markedly lessened. We take ourselves out of the vicious circles of worrying and being uptight over having the pain, which only makes the pain worse. You can also use WHEE to take the edge off the suffering of your pains, diminishing it to more tolerable levels.

As we grow through the lessons of our pains, we may find that life becomes dearer, sweeter, and more full of love. The affirmations of WHEE facilitate this wakening to deeper appreciation of what life has to offer us.

The Shadow

> *There is no light without shadow and no psychic wholeness without imperfection. To round itself out, life...calls not for perfection but for completeness; and for this the "thorn in the flesh" is needed, the suffering of defects without which there is no progress and no ascent.*

—Carl Jung

Many would include a discussion of shadow aspects of our being under psychological issues. I feel, however, that this topic belongs here, under spiritual issues, because the shadow, like pain, is an invitation from our higher self to look more deeply into the meanings of our life.

People tend to have strong preferences or inclinations in how they relate to the world: some favor the mind and outer senses, while others experience life and interact through their feelings and intuitions. People who are strong on one side of these polarities tend to be less connected with the opposite poles. Carl Jung developed extensive theories around these polarities, illustrated in the diagram of Figure 3.

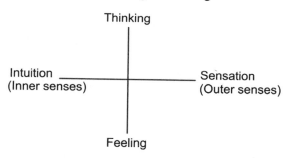

Figure 3. Jungian Polarities.

Extroverts focus on objects and people external to themselves, and experience the world as a series of interactions with these outside objects. *Introverts* are focused on their inner awareness, living their conscious lives under the influence of whichever of the four polarities are dominant in them, without becoming too tightly bound to the outer world. Within each of these Jungian polarities are varying degrees of insightfulness and wide ranges of behavior, so the basic polarities explain some but not all aspects of people's various ways of being in the world.

While each person may readily acknowledge their own primary traits, they may not be aware that their polar opposites are also alive and active in the *shadow* aspects of their being, outside of their conscious awareness. Until recently we have been encouraged to maintain cultural stereotypes of men as thinking/sensation primaries, and women as feeling/intuitive primaries. Women's liberation has transformative in helping us to acknowledge our neglected polar opposites, giving women permission and encouragement to engage and express their *thinking* and *sensation* aspects, and encouraging men to acknowledge and express their *feeling* and *intuitive* sides.

Some of my instincts tell me not to follow some of my other instincts.

—Ashleigh Brilliant

The shadow aspects of our personalities seek expression just as much as our conscious polarities do. For instance, a "thinking" primary person will also have feelings that want and need to be expressed. If the feelings are held in, they tend to build up until they find some outlet, often under conditions of pressure or stress, when the dominant polarity loses some of its control. When these repressed feelings finally do come to expression, it is often through interactions with other people that stir the shadow to strong responses. When this happens the eruption of these feelings into consciousness and their expression in words or actions often occurs in ways that are counter-productive. Explosions of emotion, in turn, often generate negative reactions. Such experiences discourage people from giving vent to their shadow sides.

Unconsciously, people commonly choose a friend or mate with opposite polar preferences for stimulation and balance, but also because they can let the other express aspects of themselves that they would rather not acknowledge or deal with. For example, a husband with primary introverted, thinking/sensation functions may be happy to see his wife with primary extroverted, intuitive/feeling functions handle decorating and social affairs at home. The wife may leave finances, car maintenance, and home repairs to her husband. Thus, each avoids engaging their shadow or *inferior* polarities. Such arrangements can work in the opposite direction as well. A feeling partner can help a thinking partner be more aware of their own feelings, and vice-versa.

If my heart could do my thinking would my brain begin to feel?

—Van Morrison

The shadow aspect of our unconscious mind also shuts away those parts of our being that make us uncomfortable, and that we would rather not acknowledge to ourselves and to others. This shadow carries all of our unacknowledged, deeply buried old hurts with their accompanying angers and resentments, as well as all the little and great envies and desires that parents and religious institutions teach us we ought not to have, though we invariably do—and more besides.

These shadow aspects of our psychological makeup are every bit as much a part of ourselves as the other aspects that are within our conscious awareness. As such, they influence our beliefs, perceptions, feelings, and actions—often completely without our conscious awareness. These are our irrational desires and fears, our un*reason*able reactions — precisely because they abide and function deep below the level of our reasoning mind. They operate outside of our *persona*—the part of our selves that we construct and groom in order to present the best possible face to ourselves and to those around us. We may become aware of our shadow parts when we catch ourselves in excessively strong outbursts of hurt or angry feelings, when we examine our dreams, or when others point out that they feel our behaviors are inappropriate.

The Pain Body

Man is sometimes extraordinarily, passionately in love with suffering.

—Fyodor Dostoevsky

The *emotional pain body*, as identified by Eckhart Tolle, is a part of ourselves that is derived from negativity that we have incorporated from unpleasant and painful experiences in our lives. The pain body is habituated or addicted to pain: it feeds on negative, distressing, painful experiences, and will provoke situations that generate these. It may be dormant for short or long periods of time, but gets triggered to activity by negative experiences that resonate with its history and patterns of distressing experiences. It may be mild and relatively harmless or it can be aggressive and self-destructive, even violent. This is the part of ourselves that creates conflicts between people who are close with each other.

Tolle's pain body sounds a lot like an aspect of what Jung describes as the shadow. I find, however, that people readily relate to their pain body, while they may have much more difficulty connecting with their shadow as a concept and as a personal awareness.

Tolle notes that the pain body shrinks with our awareness of being in the present moment, which he calls *the Now*, and with our letting go of our mental addictions to beliefs and feelings about who we are, also known as the *ego*. With time, we can learn to let the pain body go by becoming conscious of and being present with its existence, rather than moving into negativity. This will immediately start to weaken the pain body's hold on us.

Intrigued by Tolle's description of this aspect of ourselves, I decided to seek out my own pain body. In my explorations I found that it is part of my Inner Child, yet it preferred to be recognized as a distinct entity. This inner connection with the pain body made it markedly easier to clear my issues of emotional pain using WHEE, because issues are released more quickly through the Inner Child than when addressed as memories.

I recalled clearly how, as a child, I experienced my mother venting her pain body on me in periodic angry tirades that were completely out of proportion to anything I had done or not done. I would sometimes deliberately provoke her to discharge her pain body when I saw it heating up, rather than sit on the volcano until it exploded on its own.

Using WHEE with my pain body and Inner Child, I was able to clear a lot of the residuals from these experiences, five or six decades after the original traumas.

While the pain body may be a negative force in our lives, like any other pain, it may also compel us to examine our lives and to choose more healing ways of relating to ourselves, to each other, and to the world around us. One of the most common ways to become aware of our pain body is through relationships with people close to us.

Tim and Carol had been a happy couple during their two years of dating and engagement. Five months into their marriage, however, they were terribly distressed to find themselves in a series of arguments that escalated to the point of Tim becoming physically violent. Three times he promised he would never again hit Carol, yet each time they got into a heated argument he lashed out and struck her.

In couple's counseling, it was clear that they loved each other and wanted to make a go of their relationship but were unable to control their surface feelings and behaviors that led to Tim's explosions. They could see that their childhood histories held clear parallels with their current difficulties. Tim's father had been a binge drinker with an explosive temper. Tim had been terrified to go home after school on Fridays because he knew he was going to face his father's verbal and physical abuse over the weekend. Carol's father had had a pattern similar to Tim's. She was astounded to be reminded of this when we reviewed her life history. "I swore I'd never go near anyone like my dad," she said. "In the two years that Tim and I dated, he never behaved this way."

Both Carol and Tim used WHEE to clear the buried feelings in their pain bodies, including terrors, hurt, and anger from their childhood experiences. Once these had been released, and positives installed to replace them, their relationship was free of these outbursts.

I am fortunate in having easy access to my Inner Child and a cooperative response from my *Inner Hurt Child* that is the pain body. This comes from working for many years on these and other aspects of myself with WHEE and with a variety of methods. Tim and Carol had similar experiences to mine. Others may find their pain body so hurt, fearful, and angry that it is difficult to access and well defended behind meta-anxieties. Nevertheless, with patience and persistence it is possible to work our way through these resistances and to bring healing to the pain body through WHEE.

Tolle reports that the pain body can be very strong and difficult to deal with. I approach this from the opposite side, noting that many people have difficulties being firm with their Inner Child, including the pain body. When this is the case, the pain body comes to behave as a hurt, spoiled child who has managed to blackmail his or her parents with threats of various sorts, or who has become spoiled because of various other parental issues. Having studied and worked in family systems therapy, I am keenly aware of ways in which parents subtly enable and encourage children to act out the parents' hurts, angers, and other issues. When the Inner Parent is strengthened and reasons for acting out through the pain body are explored and dealt with, the pain body can be addressed more readily, fully, and competently.

In Transactional Analysis, there is also the concept of *contamination,* in which the boundaries between the Adult and the Child ego states may be poor. In effect, the Inner Adult may blend to some degree with the Child, so that the Adult doesn't even recognize we are behaving at times as a child. See Figure 4 for a diagram of this contamination. Again, this is consistent with Tolle's description of the process required for healing: the Adult must recognize the contamination and then the Child cannot get away with its misbehaviors as easily. Figure 4 shows a mild contamination, where it may be reasonably easy for the Adult portion of the person to recognize what is happening and to correct it. With more profound invasion of the Inner Adult by the Child, it may even be impossible for the Adult to recognize that this has occurred because the Child so strongly colors the Adult's awareness.

What I am saying addresses the hurt child/pain body at the levels of emotions, mind, and relationships. The behaviors of the hurt child/pain body in seeking to generate distress in other people is similar to the behaviors of children in gangs, particularly prominent in teen years. These children, often struggling to find self-empowerment in social settings fraught with racism, classism, and broken homes, seek the support

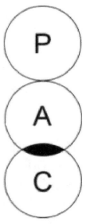

Figure 4. Contamination of the Inner Adult by the Child.

of peers. This will nearly always be far less than satisfying because their peers are just as emotionally needy and seek exactly the same nurturing. Therefore, members of gangs often are unable to provide the love and caring that each of its members is seeking. This generates a group dynamic of angers that are projected outward collectively. This enables gang members to release a small measure of their personal, individual hurts and angers indirectly—without fully connecting with the depths of their personal painful feelings.

Gang behavior is a venting of hurts that are often at the level of a post-traumatic stress disorder (PTSD). One of the characteristics of a PTSD, as mentioned earlier, is the inflicting of pains on others that are similar to the pains one experienced oneself. The psychological pain body/hurt child behaves in the very same way, but is often not recognized as venting the pent-up feelings of a buried PTSD. Families, schools, and law enforcement agencies often get caught up in the crisis and drama of the angry interactions and seek to control the behaviors, without dealing with the underlying feelings.

Tolle addresses the pain body at the energetic level. This is an extremely helpful way to understand buried pains in individuals that resonate with the pains in others. In an energetic model of this process, the combined pain of a group comes into expression through a gang's violence or a nation's collective venting of hurts and angers on "others." This discussion could have been placed in the Chapter 2 section on the unconscious mind. However, I feel that Tolle's ways of addressing the pain body through the practice of mindfulness meditation, and his observations on the collective pain body are valid and therefore belong in this chapter.

Many traditions and philosophies teach that much of our consciousness is involved in mental chatter and other preoccupations that serve to maintain our sense of individual and collective self, or ego, as a separate entity in the world. Therefore, much of our misery stems from our efforts to defend our ego and to run away from our fears of not being in control of our destiny. The truth is, we are not in control and cannot be in control, in a world that is full of uncertainties. That we experience pain as intensely unpleasant is due to our responses to the pain. If we just accept the pain, it feels much less painful. WHEE can help us release our struggles with pain and accept it.

Tolle explains that the pain body survives in our energies and consciousness from one incarnation to another. This is a part of our *karma*, the unresolved feelings and relationships that we return to work through in future lifetimes when we do not complete the clearing in the lifetime when the negativity was generated. Such residues in our pain body may be particularly challenging to deal with when we died an unhappy or violent death and did not resolve the feelings that were generated in the last moments of our lives. WHEE can be helpful in releasing past-life residues such as these.

Acceptance

> *There are three days in the week: Yesterday, Today and Tomorrow.*
>
> —Richard O'Brien

Spiritual teachings from many traditions tell us that we live in the eternal *Now*. What appear to be time-past and time-future are just mental constructs that have no real substance except in our minds. When we completely accept whatever we are experiencing in the present moment, and remain completely focused upon the Now, we do not feel distress over that which did or did not happen in the past, nor anxieties or worries about what has yet to happen in the future. Much of the unpleasantness in experiencing pain derives from memories of past pains and from anticipations of possible future suffering and consequences of the pain process. Negative memories and anticipations put us into tensions that generate perpetuate, and worsen vicious circles that then worsen the pains. By being in the Now our pains can be markedly lessened. This also frees up energies to engage in positive aspects of our lives.

> *Life might not be the party we hoped for, but while we're here we might as well dance.*
>
> —Anonymous

Being in the Now is a total engagement with whatever exists in our life in the present moment. Even judging the moment as either positive or negative distances us from the moment itself—into thinking *about* the moment rather than living it. As we deepen our practice of acceptance, we find we can relinquish all thoughts and judgments about the present.

Exercises: In his body of work Eckhart Tolle presents an enormous variety of exercises for reaching a state where we can dwell in the Now. Some examples include:

- Watch the breath move in and out by itself. With this practice, many of us are able to let go of other thoughts and worries and become totally present in the Now.

- Whenever we catch ourselves speculating about the future or rehashing the past, we can recall that only the present moment is real. Being in the moment, we connect with our true self and are authentic in what we are doing. Even thinking about the book we are walking across the room to pick up is a shift into the future; to be present in the moment we focus on walking until we reach the book, and then focus on the book.

- When we catch ourselves *in a plan of doing* rather than *being* we can let go of our goal-orientation and return to the Now. Tolle gives the examples of working with our focus on a goal, or talking with another person with an agenda in mind rather than being present with that person.

Tolle's approaches are largely cognitive. By observing ourselves diligently, and by constantly returning to the Now we gradually move towards an enlightened state. Some are fortunate and are touched by the Divine, entering a state of enlightenment in an instant. Most of us, however, gradually move into this state with a lot of hard work. In essence, Tolle's approach—which draws heavily from Buddhist philosophy and practice—is a spiritual form of cognitive behavioral therapy.

WHEE can significantly augment and shortcut the process of letting go of goal orientation and other mental habits that divert us from the Now. Experiment with the following statements, or create your own:

- "Even though I dearly want to [finish this job/do whatever I need to do to hold onto this relationship/attain this goal], I still love and accept myself…"

- "Even though thoughts from the past [about "x"] intrude when I am meditating…"

- "Even though I am [frustrated/discouraged/angry with myself] for my slow progress in [mindfulness/meditation/other practices]..."

While Tolle recommends these practices for everyone, my experience as a therapist and teacher of wholistic healing is that people with strong thinking and intuitive facilities (in terms of Jungian polarities illustrated in Figure 3) do best with such an approach; those who are strong in feeling and outer senses may need a lot of support. For instance, Tolle suggests that people with addictions to alcohol or other substances could refocus on the Now as a way of dealing with cravings. While this may help on the milder end of the addictions spectrum, or in later stages of 12-step practices, I know of very few who can use mindfulness in the initial stages of dealing with addictions.

It can be quite a stretch for those of us raised in Western culture to grasp the wisdom and value of staying in the Now and not pushing ourselves to achieve goals. In fact, it appears to many who are considering practices of being in the Now that these could derail them from achieving success in their careers and life-paths. Tolle advises that it is just the opposite. When we are totally present in the Now, we are more than intimately connected with our true self. We *are* our true self. This will further our life purpose more than any goal-directed planning and behaviors. We will be in the flow of the collective consciousness as well as being in our own flow. The following apocryphal story from the Zen tradition illustrates this point:

> A poor farmer in China had a single horse. This horse was essential to his work. It pulled his plow, brought his produce to market, and provided transportation for his family.
>
> One day, the farmer woke to find the gate open and the horse gone. His neighbors came around to commiserate with him over his loss. He responded only with, "We'll see."
>
> Two days later, his stallion returned with a herd of 20 wild mares. His neighbors came around to congratulate him on his wonderful good fortune. Again, he responded only with, "We'll see."
>
> The next day, his only son was struggling to ride one of the wild mares and broke his leg. His neighbors came around

again to commiserate with him over his bad luck. Again, he responded only with, "We'll see."

A week later, the local warlord came to their village, drafting every able-bodied young male for his army. Naturally, he was unable to take the farmer's son. His neighbors came around again to congratulate him on his wonderful good fortune. Yet again, he responded only with, "We'll see."

Our understanding of reality in any given moment is based on limited awareness of the larger picture. In the fullness of time, we come to appreciate that what we comprehended about a situation may have been partly or totally erroneous, based on the facts we had available for our consideration at the time. Nearly all of our analyses and fretting about our current moment end up for naught—other than to provide chewing gum for the mind. In hindsight, we might even begin to appreciate that an apparent misfortune or even a tragedy turns out to have life-transforming benefits for us.

When we accept what *is* and don't fret over what isn't, our lives can be much more peaceful and satisfying. This doesn't mean we abandon all planning and goal-directed activities, but rather that we don't attach expectations to specific outcomes. I cannot count the times the Chinese farmer principle has proven itself in my own life.

For example, I grumbled at my mother for many years about pushing me to go to medical school, and at myself for having accepted her advice. I was working as a psychotherapist, after having trained in psychiatry. This had required a total of eight years' training. I felt that much of what I had learned in medical school and internship (five of the eight years) had been a waste of my time. The psychiatric training in those days was nearly all focused on psychotherapy, and I had some outstanding teachers and role models, so I didn't complain about that part of my education. But I much preferred the psychotherapy to prescribing tranquilizing and antidepressant medications, which slowly became the primary focus of my job expectations as a psychiatrist.

As I moved into exploring wholistic spiritual healing, however, my medical credentials gave me more credibility than I would otherwise have received as a psychotherapist with a degree in counseling, social work, or psychology. At that point, I became grateful that I had followed my mother's advice and urgings.

In another instance, I was distressed and disappointed when we had to cancel a week and a half of workshops in South Korea due to low registrations. Only a few years earlier, I most likely would have put myself through great anxiety, recriminations over decisions of commission or omission, analyses of what I might have done differently to prevent the cancellation, and so on. I am pleased and relieved that this sort of painful cogitation is lessening, as I learn to live more in the present and accept what is as the reality of my now, not putting myself through a wringer over what I could have done differently or what might happen as consequences in the future.

A week later, it turned out that my presence at home was needed in a major project that was more important to me than the trip abroad. A research grant application to study WHEE and related methods needed intensive work on several fronts just at the time I would have been traveling. The university where the study was to be run phoned to say they had reversed their agreement to let us proceed with their review board. Without this approval, the grant application was in jeopardy. Several days later — the day prior to my previously programmed departure — one of the therapists who had committed to providing therapy in the study resigned due to overwork. At the same time, several excellent suggestions arrived from colleagues for strengthening the research proposal. All of this occurred at the last minute for amending the grant application for this study. Had I been abroad, there is a strong chance the study would have faltered and would have had to be postponed.

Muscle testing has been extremely useful in these recurrent lessons on what I have fondly come to call "the big P and T" (patience and trust). My left-brain logic continues to question my inner gnowing of the rightness of the flow of life. I ask transpersonal questions such as, "Will it be for my highest good and the highest good of all to [anticipate there are positive sides to what is happening that will soon become apparent/continue with the research project even though it appears it is falling apart/trust that the time I am committing to this project will bear fruit that will justify this personal investment]?"

The unfolding of the outcomes to these challenges then either validates the inner gnowing and muscle testing, or provides corrective feedback on my process of using it. The same day the therapist resigned, we found a replacement therapist who felt more compatible with the research study, and found a colleague who was able to promise help with research board approval plus much further help with data analysis and writeups required for all phases of the study. I must admit that I had a very difficult time remembering the Chinese Farmer and not rushing to cheer loudly!

These aspects of acceptance highlight our participation in collective consciousness, confirming Eckhart Tolle's predictions that when we are in the Now our life purpose manifests and brings us into the flow, where we participate with others in a cosmic dance, choreographed by an unseen but ever-present Producer.[16]

Love and Compassion

Love and compassion are necessities, not luxuries. Without them humanity cannot survive.

—His Holiness The Dalai Lama

I had a very wise supervisor in my first year of psychiatric residency training. He said, "If you can't find something you love about the person you're treating, it's better not to be treating them."

Love is a vital element in any therapeutic encounter, as unconditional positive regard of one person for another is a palpable force for healing. This essential element has been missing in the lives of many people who come for therapy. By sensing the therapist's love, they find within themselves that which can open to being loved by others.

The English language is a poor one for discussing love, as there are no separate words to distinguish between the love we feel for a spouse, parent, child, or other family member and love for a person who is under our therapeutic care or for our country, a particular food or other pleasurable experience, and so on. Still, there are distinct qualitative differences between these that are palpable to anyone who gives them some thought. I point this out just to be absolutely clear that I am not suggesting that those who practice WHEE (or any other type of therapists) should become romantically involved with their clients.

---

[16] Much more on deeper understandings of spiritual reality in *Healing Research, Volume 3, Personal Spirituality* and in the *Personal Spirituality Workbook*.

*Love. It is the only choice. And the opposite of dying is not living—
but is love; the opposite of love (and life) is not death—it is fear; and the
constriction of life that causes. Death is not the end of life. But fear can
close off love—and the worst fear of all is the fear of love, itself.*

— Mary Ann Wallace

To help people on the deepest possible levels using WHEE, love
must be present—as with any other therapy. What is particularly helpful in this regard as it pertains to WHEE, however, is that anything
negative that is roused or triggered in therapists by their clients can be
cleared with the technique. This can therefore eliminate most blocks or
impediments to therapists feeling love for their clients.

Compassion is the understanding and appreciation of another
person's emotional state and the wish to lessen or alleviate that person's
suffering. Compassion opens us to feeling empathy for that person and
to "do unto others that which we would have them do unto us."

WHEE is always taught to therapists experientially, so that they
can connect with their own pains. This helps them to empathize with
clients who are in physical or psychological pain, and to offer treatment
compassionately.

Forgiveness

*The more grudges you carry, the heavier your burden becomes.
Forgive, and let them go. When someone has wronged you, it hurts. There
is certainly no sense in using your own time and energy to prolong that
hurt. Forgive, and you can begin to move away from the pain. Forgive,
and you can move forward with a much lighter load.... Forgive, and
you'll be much better off. Forgive, and you'll be free to truly live.*

— Ralph Marston

The pain of feeling that we have been hurt by others may be one of
the most difficult injuries to deal with. This is especially true when those
who hurt us were members of our family or close friends who we would
have hoped and expected to treat us with caring love and compassion.

I have seen countless people who were able to clear major physical
and psychological pains associated with severe injuries from automobile
accidents, assaults, rapes, and medical practice misfortunes. They were

able to release pains; fears; anxieties about re-injuries; grief over disfigurement, losses of body parts and functions; broken trust, and betrayals in long-term, close relationships; angers at those responsible for their pains and injuries, as well as at medical, police, emergency services, legal, judiciary and penal personnel and institutions whom they felt treated them unfairly, incompetently or unjustly.

One of the last pieces of work required in many experiences of releasing issues with WHEE is often that of forgiveness. Even having released all of the issues above, plus more individual and personal issues that extend beyond that woeful list, a simmering element of resentment remained:

- "Okay, so he was drunk when he was driving after the Christmas party and hit me in the crosswalk, leaving me paralyzed from the waist down, with brain injuries and terrible headaches. I keep thinking that a year in jail in no way compensates me for what he destroyed in my life."

- "I'm no longer angry, because that just hurts me in the end. But I am still deeply bothered that my father was so insensitive and uncaring about me that he would satisfy his sex drive using my body—as though I were not there as a person, much less his daughter."

- "I feel like God must be punishing me by giving me this [pain/injury/disease/misfortune], so how could I say, 'God loves and accepts me?'"

Hardest of all may be the challenge of forgiving oneself for contributing to whatever happened. We tend to be our own worst critics!

- "If only I had been more alert to the traffic instead of fumbling with my gift packages as I crossed the street when I was hit by that drunk driver."

- "If only I had talked to my [mother/other family member/pastor/teacher/counselor] about what my father was doing to me, I wouldn't have been as messed up as I am today."

- "If I hadn't ignored what my [parents/family/church] taught me, I wouldn't have all this pain and suffering."

It is easier for many people to let go of other bothersome feelings than to let go of their resentments. WHEE makes it easier to work on forgiveness through the immediate feedback people have from releasing other feelings. They learn that they feel so much better emotionally and that their physical and psychological pains are markedly lessened when they release these negative feelings. They can then perceive that they may feel better yet if they release whatever resentments hold them back from forgiving the person whom they feel has wronged or injured them.

Once the commitment is made to work on forgiveness, WHEE can help to release whatever negative feelings are preventing a person from reaching that goal. In some instances, residuals of hurt, fear, or anger are discovered to have been previously blocking forgiveness. In other cases, the difficulties in forgiving can be addressed directly with WHEE: "Even though I feel it is hard for me to forgive…."

Forgiveness is an issue where it is generally helpful to move slowly and to carefully record the exact words used. If resistances block progress, the words we use will often provide clues to the issues that can be addressed.

Forgiving is not forgetting. It is remembering and letting go.

—Claudia Black

I have never regretted my decision to study and practice psychotherapy. My work with others and on myself is a never-ending series of wonderful lessons and awakenings into ever-deeper appreciation for the wonder of being alive.

I peeled many layers of the onion of my hurts and angers from my relationship with my mother, but for years after she had died I was still unable to come to a place of forgiveness over her inability to see and accept me for myself. Even though I had come to understand that her self-centeredness was due to the hurts she herself had experienced in childhood, and even though I used every variation of WHEE I could muster, the resentments remained. I simply was not able to forgive and forget.

In addressing other layers of my onion, I worked with my Inner Child, promising that I would spend time with Little Dan daily. I meant it sincerely when I made the promise, but my mild ADHD distractibility led me to overlook many times that I could have invited Little Dan to participate in playful or joyful activities.

In asking forgiveness from Little Dan, I realized that my insensitivity to his needs and my broken promises to make amends were very similar to my mother's behaviors toward me. In working on forgiving myself, I was then able to come into a place of forgiving my mother.

There is certainly a wonderful feeling of release with forgiveness — of oneself as well as of others.

❧

Transcending Pain

He who learns must suffer, and, even in our sleep, pain that cannot forget falls drop by drop upon the heart, and in our own despair, against our will, comes wisdom to us by the awful grace of God.

—Aeschylus

Pain is a challenge we can rarely ignore. When we have suffered with it for a while, any relief we obtain is a blessing and full relief may feel like a miracle. When we have transcended our pain with WHEE, there is a tremendous relief of suffering. There are often great enhancements of awareness at the same time: connecting with levels of our being and deepening connections that we may not even have been aware were there; learning to listen to our inner wisdom and higher selves; and gaining empathy for the suffering of others.

Some conditions of pain may not release entirely. In such cases, WHEE can be helpful in dealing with our meta-issues of anxieties, distress, and disappointments at having to deal with chronic pain. Activity, imagery, hypnotic, and distraction techniques can also help to move the awareness of pain into the background of our consciousness. They all work on the principle that if we focus on the pain, it intensifies; if we focus elsewhere, it fades into the background and may even disappear.[17] WHEE can help to strengthen these approaches through installing positives of imagery, focus, and intent. For instance:

- "I can ignore my pain and focus on [pleasant image/memory/music] and I love and accept myself…"

- "I can deeply and completely immerse myself in [favorite activity] and I…"

---

[17] See suggestions in Caudill; Cohen; Rossi, Turk; Zeig.

Additionally, many complementary and alternative therapies can help to alleviate chronic pain, including acupuncture and its derivatives, Chinese medicine, and electrical nerve stimulation.[18]

Pain as Teacher

If we allow our pain to be felt and freed, our suffering does great work in softening our hearts. It is, in the words of Trungpa Rinpoche, "manure for the field of wisdom." In fact, it is important to know that any difficult mind state is welcome to arise at any moment just as the sky welcomes whatever arises in it without resistance. Our suffering, if we feel it deeply and allow its natural passing, makes us stronger and yet more tender. We are whole not only despite what we have suffered but often because of it.

—Catherine Ingram

Pain is a challenge that can either wear people down or invite them to shift to new life paths and rise to heights they had not known were possible. WHEE can help on either path. As Viktor Frankl said, "What is to give light must endure burning."

At first it may be difficult to even conceive of the possibility of relating to pain in any way other than as a scourge to be avoided whenever feasible, and to be diminished through whatever means possible. This is a natural reaction, often born of many experiences that were stressful, hurtful, and frustrating—because we did not have tools like WHEE to deal with our pains and found them to be unpleasant and perhaps even overwhelming.

As WHEE helps us let go of old habits of responding to pain with distress, annoyance, frustration, anxieties, fears, and anger, a space opens up for us to relate very differently to our pain. As we dialogue with our pains and our pain body, as we gain confidence in being able to understand our pains, and as we feel confident in dealing with them, our attitudes can shift. With a more tolerant, even positive attitude toward our pains, we can greet them as we might greet any teacher—with respect, patience, and openness to learning what they offer to teach. We are then well on our way to firming up a sweetening spiral in our lives, building from one success to another.

---

[18] These and numerous other approaches are reviewed, with extensive references, in *Healing Research, Volumes 2.*

7

Theories to Explain WHEE

The good physician treats the disease; the great physician treats the patient who has the disease.

—Hippocrates

L et us first look at practical explanations for why WHEE works so well to relieve pains and stress. Then, once the foundation has been laid, we may better understand the speculations on deeper questions raised by these transformative processes.

Process and Content Explanations

Learn to get in touch with silence within yourself, and know that everything in this life has purpose. There are no mistakes, no coincidences. All events are blessings given to us to learn from.

—Elizabeth Kübler-Ross

WHEE is successful beyond any other therapy I have ever used, for myself and for my clients. In great part, this is due to specific factors of wholistic understanding and approaches, combined with the procedures included in WHEE.

- WHEE is technically simple. Everyone can learn the basic procedure in less than ten minutes.

- WHEE is elegantly simple, allowing for applications on a wide variety of problems, addressing them at many levels of their complexities.

- WHEE's rapidity allows for much greater flexibility in working on target problems within the session.

- WHEE is highly individualized to suit each person's specific needs and preferences.

- WHEE is constantly tweaked and adapted to the specific issues of each user, as the process unfolds, with sharpening of focus and refinements in the elements selected for WHEE work.

- WHEE addresses every level of one's being.

- WHEE's practical focus on releasing old patterns and installing new ones wherever trauma and blocks are found is highly effective.

- WHEE introduces small, incremental changes that enable users to identify immediately the specific components that work well for them.

- WHEE makes it easy to explore underlying issues and alternative methods of addressing them when a person has difficulties in lightening their pains and other problems.

- WHEE is very well accepted and compliance outside the therapy room is much higher because of its simplicity.

- WHEE is tremendously empowering, as it is so simple and so rapidly effective in self-healing. People are very pleased to be able to help themselves, not having to rely constantly on medications or the interventions of a therapist, although with challenging situations the guidance of a therapist can markedly facilitate the self-healing uses of WHEE.

- WHEE provides a method for decreasing anxieties and fears as soon as they arise—in clients and therapists. With time, a sweetening spiral develops: success in dealing with fears → confidence in dealing with fears → facing fears as soon as they become conscious → more success in dealing with fears. Therapists and clients no longer run away from or avoid facing their fears, which markedly facilitates therapy.

- WHEE invites us to connect more deeply with our spiritual awareness.

I have been exploring complementary/alternative therapies (CAM) for close to forty years, after studying psychology, medicine, psychiatry, and research. My studies have not been superficial, as testified by the weighty tomes of *Healing Research, Volumes 1–3.*

In studying and implementing these wide varieties of helpful approaches, I have gleaned numerous ways to facilitate self-healing on all levels of one's being. Much of the success of WHEE resides in its addressing people's problems along the entire wholistic spectrum from body through spirit. Though each aspect of WHEE may have its initial focus on one level, it often interconnects with the other levels in the unfolding of the therapy process.

Putting this in wholistic terms, WHEE addresses the entire person and not just the symptoms of dis-ease or disease the person presents as a focus for treatment. Most people readily accept and appreciate this approach. Some people may identify their problem as one of emotional (or other wholistic level) distress and when invited to explore other levels, may ask, "Why are we wandering so far away from the problem?" They may feel more comfortable if the wholistic approach is explained.

Let's proceed with a review of the many ways WHEE can be helpful. While this discussion dissects the component levels of the wholistic spectrum, you will readily appreciate that in many cases each piece is intimately linked with pieces and aspects of other levels.

Body

> And your body is the harp of your soul,
> It is yours to bring forth sweet music from it or confused sounds.
> And forget not that the earth delights to feel your bare feet
> And the winds longs to play with your hair.

—Kahlil Gibran

The body is intimately interlinked with emotions and mind. Many are now referring to this unity as the mind-body or bodymind. By inviting the body to participate in releasing negatives and installing positives, we strengthen and deepen a person's responses to WHEE.

Here are ways the body participates in stress, pain, and other symptoms, and how it responds to the wholistic healing of WHEE:

- Feeling memories are stored as a matter of course in the body. This seems particularly true of traumatic experiences.

- When we repeat metaphoric expressions such as, "What a headache this is!" or "I'm getting butterflies in my stomach!" we program our body to be tense in the parts we mention in our metaphors. This sensitizes particular regions of our body to later go into spasm or in other ways speak to us, since we have unconsciously linked them to particular issues of stress or other negativity.

- Our body can answer our inner questions and speak to us if we invite it to tell us what it wants us to know about our symptoms, illnesses, and unconscious processes.

- Our body will often monitor our promises to change and our progress in doing so—reminding us, if necessary, of our commitments through intensifying our pain and other symptoms.

- Our body can be an instrument for further communications with our unconscious mind through muscle testing.

- Our body's immune system is closely connected with our thought and feeling processes, and can be activated to deal with relevant aspects of immune diseases.

The body helps us to understand where we are in life. It can connect us with deeper layers of physical and psychological issues that contribute to pain and dis-ease, particularly when we dialogue with parts of our body that are complaining through pain or illness, and when we use muscle testing. Whatever we uncover in these intimate and revealing discussions with our unconscious mind may then be addressed through rounds of WHEE to release negativity and install replacement positives.

As we learn to use muscle testing, we strengthen our abilities to access our intuition. This opens us to connect more consciously and more strongly through our bodymind with our existence as energy beings and with extrasensory perceptions, the collective consciousness, and personal spiritual awareness, thereby vastly expanding and deepening the range of our self-healing capacities.

Coming from the opposite direction, as we deliberately explore our intuitive capacities, we get feedback as to the accuracy of our muscle testing. This helps to bridge the conceptual divides that Western scientific approaches have built into our self-awareness through labeling and studying each of the subsections of the wholistic spectrum in isolation from the others.

In these ways, body connects with mind, emotions, relationships, and spirit.

Emotions

There can be no transforming of darkness into light and of apathy into movement without emotion.

—Carl Jung

Emotions are a major portion of the language we use in our interactions with our inner selves, as well as in our relationships with other people and the greater world around us. We may feel hurt, anxious, fearful, angry, or sad in response to negative events in our lives; or we may feel joy, happiness, peace, compassion, love, and elation with positive experiences. The particular emotions that come forth depend on our personality, mood, type, intensity and past experiences with similar situations and relationships, anticipations surrounding the circumstances, and much more.

Strong emotional responses in our present lives—in ourselves and in the responses we experience from others—are stimuli to explore our past experiences and our inner rules about relating to people. When we follow these clues and do the detective work invited by our unconscious mind, we often awaken to see and hear others as they really are, uncover inner fears that block us from being present, and reassess how we may be responding according to inner rules we established long ago for handling our emotions, rather than being in the Now.

WHEE provides a tool for softening emotions that are negative and/or uncomfortable, and for installing positive emotions to replace those we have released. WHEE is powerful in dealing with emotions because:

- Using the SUDS and SUSS sensitizes people to the fine nuances of intensity in their emotions. This can help people who have previously not been in touch with their feelings to make the connection.

- As we use WHEE, we experience shifts in SUDS and SUSS that give us feedback on how effective the WHEE process is for dealing with emotions, even when they may have been troublesome for a long time. This neutralizes much of the fear we carry from child-hood programming about not letting our hurt feelings surface to consciousness.

- WHEE tracks emotions constantly to ensure that the self-healing remains as sharply focused as possible, adjusting and adapting the statement of the problem focus as you proceed.

- WHEE strongly recommends reducing the SUDS all the way to zero if at all possible, in order to complete the releasing process with a given emotional focus.

- When we encounter resistances to releasing emotions, WHEE provides immediate ways to identify and address the meta-issues or past issues that will then release the blocks.

- WHEE enables the installation of positives after releasing the negatives.

- Positives may also be installed when we are depressed, blocked by resistances, or in distress or despair over the opening of old, buried issues.

- Using WHEE over a period of time instills confidence that it is pos-sible to deal constructively with any emotions we wish to address.

- The confidence gained in the abilities to handle emotions makes it possible to respond to new situations with a lower intensity of emotional reactivity, because we are not as likely to get into meta-anxieties or other meta-issues of being worried that we might be overwhelmed by our emotions.

- With the growing confidence of repeated successes with WHEE, sweetening spirals are developed. When troubling emotions are aroused, they come to be viewed as invitations to clear old, underly-ing issues as well as the current upset.

- WHEE is closely and carefully tailored to suit individual needs and is not prescriptive in how to deal with emotional issues. This leads people to experience WHEE as a very accepting and affirming modality.

In all these ways, WHEE facilitates the development of emotional intelligence, which I define as the harmonious blending of mind with emotions.

Being able to enter flow is emotional intelligence at its best; flow represents perhaps the ultimate in harnessing the emotions in the service of performance and learning. In flow the emotions are not just contained and channeled, but positive, energized, and aligned with the task at hand.

—Daniel Goleman

If we live either through mind or emotions alone, our lives are often skewed to the point of being dysfunctional. We were given both facilities in our on-board computers: our emotions-focused right brain and our thinking-focused left brain hemispheres. WHEE helps to bring us into balance through the alternating right and left tapping and through working systematically on our thoughts and feelings to release negatives and install positives. Going deeper, as discussed below, WHEE also helps us open into better relationships and into deeper connections with our spiritual awareness.

Mind

The universe is transformation; our life is what our thoughts make it.

—Marcus Aurelius

Mind is where many of us live. We have all sorts of beliefs about who we are and what the world is about. These are stories and lessons we have accepted from life experiences, garnished with the teachings of our parents, schoolteachers, clergy, and the media. We tend to maintain our belief systems about who we are and how the world is held together even in the face of events and information that contradict them. It is easier to reject evidence that does not match our worldview than to change our beliefs.

Western society teaches, supports, and reinforces these mental ways of dealing with the world. We see this even in the Jungian and complementary/alternative therapies communities.

- Most Jungians focus on the feelings pole primarily as it relates to values that are held as tenets of belief—held as elementary axioms of life; known with an inner knowing that is beyond logical reasoning. My own experience, personally and as a therapist, is that the

feeling pole is readily acknowledged by most people as better relating to emotions (to contrast with the thinking pole).

- Most complementary/alternative therapists advertise that they
focus on "body, mind, and spirit." The links between body and
psychological processes have been emphasized as mind-body or
bodymind issues. Feelings and emotions may also be subjects for
focus in these therapies, but they are not mentioned.

Science holds that beliefs must be based on logical, systematic studies of the world and readjusted in the light of new evidence. The major-
ity of scientists, however, just like you and me, tend to reject evidence
that contradicts their current theories.

Scientists are trained to have strong thinking capacities and the
ability to study and manipulate the outer, material world. These people
may have difficulties connecting with and appreciating feelings and
intuitions—in themselves and in others. Rather than examine their discomforts in these areas, which in many ways may contradict their theories and beliefs of how the world works, it is easier for them to reject
and belittle whatever is involved with feelings and intuitions.

Favoring our mental analyses of the world has in large part gotten
us into the troubles we are experiencing today. We are exhibiting a
gross lack of concern for our environment, over-exploiting our resources, and polluting the planet. Within a few years, we may make Earth
uninhabitable to life as we know it.

On a personal level, the challenge for mind is to sift and sort information about our outer and inner situations and then to make response
choices that will be in our best interests. This is far more complex than
it may seem at first glance. The mind sifts and sorts whatever our senses
pick up externally. This is usually the easy part. Internally, the mind
must identify and deal with ordinary ebbs and flows of emotions, as well
as screening exaggerated, distorted, or distancing emotions.

It is even more challenging for the mind to deal with its own cus-
tomary responses that get it in trouble. As we observe ourselves in conflict with other people or get upset with ourselves, we begin to realize
that we may have problems in our thinking and imagination that also
need attention. These may be due to outmoded residues and habits from
childhood programming or from later experience residues along our
way to present-day situations.

WHEE is marvelous for helping us deal with distressing issues that bother our mind. Just as WHEE can reduce the intensity of negative emotions and install replacement positives, it can do the same with thoughts that we find troublesome. This can be very helpful with a variety of pain issues.

People appreciate WHEE for sorting out mental processes because:

- WHEE is very easy to learn and apply to all sorts of problems.

- WHEE is excellent under stress situations because it is so simple and quick that people do not get flustered to the point they can't remember how to do it.

- WHEE is flexible and adaptable to everyone's beliefs and preferences, and can be focused specifically to deal with any issues.

- WHEE takes resistances as potential clues to further issues, often releasing problems on deeper levels—rather than just focusing on resistances as blocks to be overcome on the path to getting the SUDS or SUSS to change around a symptom such as a specific pain, anxiety, or distress.

- WHEE readily identifies meta-issues and very quickly releases them, so that the primary issues can then be unblocked and released.

- When meta-issues do not respond, we can often identify core beliefs that can then be addressed with WHEE.

- WHEE quickly transforms what look at first like overwhelming worries and distressing circumstances into manageable concerns.

- As emotions that could be problematic arise, our past experiences with WHEE enable us to recognize that we have a range of options. Responses of fear, worry, anger, or other potentially problematic emotions and reactions to pain may in many cases become choices rather than reflexive responses.

- WHEE opens and deepens awareness of our intimate connections with other levels of the wholistic spectrum.

All of these benefits of WHEE make it a powerful wholistic healing tool for dealing with pains across the entire physical and psychological spectrum.

Pain makes man think. Thought makes man wise. Wisdom makes life endurable.

—John Patrick

Finding the balance between emotions, including compassion, and our conscious thinking about our inner and outer worlds may be a challenge. This is particularly true when we are working to enhance aspects of our awareness and relationships that have been neglected to the point of withering away into atrophy. When we have invested most of our lives in left-brained thinking and analyzing, it may feel overwhelming to connect with our emotions. When we have lived within our own emotional boundaries and start to reach out to connect with others on a larger scale, again we may feel overwhelmed and may need to activate our thinking capacities to sort out our inner and outer situations. WHEE can greatly facilitate the process of working out these issues, and can help us to achieve the openness and balance that allow us to be truly present. As Ram Dass wrote:

> The hardest state to be in is one in which you keep your heart open to the suffering that exists around you, and simultaneously keep your discriminative wisdom…. Once you understand that true compassion is the blending of the open heart and quiet mind, it is still difficult to find the balance. Most often we start out doing these things sequentially. We open our hearts and get lost in the melodramas, then we meditate and regain our quiet center by pulling back in from so much openness. Then we once again open and get sucked back into the dance.
>
> So it goes, cycle after cycle. It takes a good while to get the balance…. You have to stay right on the edge of that balance. It seems impossible, but you can do it. At first, when you achieve this balance, it is self-consciously maintained. Ultimately, however, you merely become the statement of the amalgam of the open heart and the quiet mind. Then there is no more struggle; it's just the way you are.

Mind also has the challenge of sifting and sorting our different experiences of intuitive awareness. Our unconscious mind scans the cosmos through telepathy, clairsentience, pre- and retrocognition, collective consciousness, and spiritual awareness, yet the perceptions it collects are often difficult to translate into concepts we can comprehend. These perceptions often surface to our conscious awareness as images that are very similar to dreams, with a richness of imagery and metaphor that invite layered explorations for ever-deeper understanding. These materials are then a challenge for us to interpret.

Relationships with Other People

In all situations, it is my response that decides whether a crisis is escalated or de-escalated, and a person is humanized or de-humanized. If we treat people as they are, we make them worse. If we treat people as they ought to be, we help them become what they are capable of becoming.

—Johann Wolfgang von Goethe

It is in our relationships that we often discover our unique child programs, and the additions and amendments we have made through the years, which we have kept without conscious awareness. We suddenly become aware of the poorly designed basic habits that contribute to or cause conflicts in our lives—both in our interactions with others and in our own inner worlds of being and behaving. When our automatic pilot programs do not match the programs of our partners, friends, and colleagues, it becomes obvious to all that we have to re-examine our basic assumptions.

Our romantic relationships can be particularly instructive in these regards. We commonly do not notice or may overlook these issues in the courting and honeymoon periods (or following the early period after moving in to live together without marrying). In the early glow of finding a compatible partner, we focus on our loving and caring exchanges. Gradually, as we explore the blending of our individual habits and routines, we find minor and major rubs. We have to change or compromise our ways of seeing and doing things in order to harmonize with the incompatibilities that are uncovered between ourselves and our partner.

Paula and Cindi had gotten along wonderfully well over several years of dating. When they moved in to live together, however, they were terribly distressed to find that their harmonious relationship seemed to be crumbling over a series of minor issues that had never bothered them before. It was the return of Cindi's migraine headaches that prompted them to seek help.

For example, Cindi was livid in her complaints about Paula's regularly leaving coffee cups around their home, and dirty dishes in the sink, and even more about Paula's neglecting to clean the tub after a bath. Paula was seriously irritated by Cindi's frequently finishing off food and kitchen items such as milk, coffee, or soap and not at least adding these to the shopping list, if not replacing them. Each had many more complaints, but these were the ones each chose to raise for sorting out in the first therapy session.

It turned out that these surface issues were not really as troublesome as the buried hurts from the past that each carried, which were stirred by the other's behaviors. Paula uncovered piles of buried anxieties, hurts, and resentments over her father's alcoholism. This had left her family in dire straits at times, even having to rely on church charity to have enough food for the children. Cindi's negligence in making sure food items were replaced was resonating with the old hurts, leading Paula to release her long buried resentments (unconsciously) onto her partner.

Cindi was the oldest of eight children and had had to help out her mother, not only because of the number of children in the family, but because her mother suffered from severe, incapacitating headaches. Paula's negligence was stirring a truckload of buried feelings from Cindi's resentments over being parentified at a very early age, having to do much of the cleaning and child rearing of her younger sisters and brothers. Cindi's migraines were probably due in part to hereditary factors and in part to festering angers and resentments that spoke out through her body. Her headaches cleared as she released the old, buried feelings in a series of WHEE sessions.

Once the underlying issues were dealt with, bundled with the current frustrations that had triggered them, Paula and Cindi found their relationship enormously more harmonious. They also noted they had greater understanding and compassion for each other and for themselves through doing these clearings.

Frustrations, resentments, hurts and angers that have been present in couples' relationships for many months and years have been successfully cleared with WHEE. These experiences illustrate how relationships help to bring out buried issues, how WHEE can help to clear the buried feelings and current issues, and how the process of couples working on their issues can bring them closer together.

Our children are shaped by our relationships with them. How we deal with the challenges, lessons, joys, and pains in our lives will be among the most important lessons they learn. Conversely, our children may be among our best teachers — bringing us through their relationships with us to re-examine on many levels how we think, feel, and relate to them, to ourselves, and to the world at large.

WHEE can aid us in dealing with reactions to our children that we feel are too strong or weak, too angry or passive, too similar or deliberately different from those of our own parents. WHEE can help our children, as well, to deal with reactions that make them uncomfortable. Merging with spiritual dimensions, emotional scars and residues can also be left by past-life relationships. Many of the examples in this book have illustrated these issues, and we will go into further detail on this last topic shortly.

Relationships with the Environment

Healing the wounds of the earth and its people does not require saintliness or a political party, only gumption and persistence. It is not a liberal or conservative activity; it is a sacred act.

— Paul Hawken

WHEE is helpful in treating animal, pollen, food, and chemical sensitivities. I have seen people with single allergies as well as multiple allergies syndrome improve tremendously with WHEE. These allergies often produce pains, including headaches and stomach cramps, and contribute to fibromyalgia.

WHEE also contributes to our broader relationships with the environment. Each of us is a part of Gaia, our planet. Each of us participates through our physical interactions and energies in what happens to our Mother Earth, who gives life to every living thing on her surface. While our single contributions to these interactions may be so minute as to seem insignificant, when we combine many grains of sand we have a beach; when we carelessly discard wastes we have pollution; and when many come together to better our Earth we have planetary healing.

As we use WHEE for intuitive awareness of our inner issues, we grow more comfortable with the range of information we can access. The feedback we get through muscle testing increases our confidence and trust in our inner knowing of what is helpful or harmful, facilitating or obstructing our growth and progress. Simlarly, when we extend the uses of WHEE to proxy/surrogate healing, we get feedback on our abilities to access intuitive/extra-sensory perception types of knowledge from outside ourselves. In validating that we can effectively send healing to other people from a distance, we confirm that we are able to influence others through these forms of interaction. We confirm that we and other people participate in a collective consciousness.

Using muscle testing for interactions with non-human parts of the world, we can confirm our interconnections with the plants, animals, waters, and atmosphere surrounding the earth:

- In considering interactions with the broader world (such as going out to the theater, a new restaurant, or on a holiday), ask yourself ahead of time, "Will I enjoy this activity?"

- When you want to spend some time outdoors and the weather is "iffy," use muscle testing to ask, "Will there be unpleasantly heavy [rains/winds] while I am outside today?"

- Uncertain about a new or potential personal or business relationship? Ask questions about the person involved. Be certain to write these down, as the way you ask the questions will influence the answers. With complex questions such as these, you may wish to repeat the process several times, as the relationship is explored and you sharpen your awareness of the questions to ask.

People in traditional cultures take intuition for granted. Their shamans can walk through nature, holding their intent that the plants and minerals needed for healing a particular person or animal will draw the shaman's attention and make themselves known. In mainstream Western cultures, our knowing is as limited by our disbeliefs in our intuitive abilities as by any innate deficits in intuitive gifts.

No Sierra landscape that I have seen holds anything truly dead or dull, or any trace of what in manufactories is called rubbish or water; everything is perfectly clean and pure and full of divine lessons. This quick, inevitable interest attaching to everything seems marvelous until the hand of God become visible; then it seems reasonable that what interests Him may well interest us. When we try to pick out anything by itself, we find it hitched to everything else in the universe.

—John Muir

As we learn this level of our interconnection with the All, we begin to appreciate that we are part of Gaia in the same way that a cell in any organ or tissue in our body is a part of ourselves. Gaia is then essential to our wellbeing in a much more direct and intimate way than is commonly appreciated.

Strengthening our awareness of Gaia and our care for her welfare is vitally important at this moment in the history of life on our planet. At present, human beings could be seen as a cancer on the planet, growing in numbers that are unchecked; consuming vital resources at rates that will soon deplete them; wantonly polluting the environment and poisoning people, animals, plants and other organisms. Rose Elizabeth Bird spoke to the devastating impact of humanity on the natural world when she said, "We have probed the earth, excavated it, burned it, ripped things from it, buried things in it....That does not fit my definition of a good tenant. If we were here on a month-to-month basis, we would have been evicted long ago."

As we release our anxieties, fears, angers and hurts on the one side, and as we strengthen our love for ourselves in our WHEE affirmations, we also enhance our capacities to relate in more loving ways with others—including Gaia.

Spirit

Our minds do and always will emotionally speculate on the unknowable, on what lies behind nature, the mysterious and miraculous adjustments conditioning all things. We shall never know, never find out, and this is what constitutes "the glory and poetry of God."

—John Galsworthy

WHEE confirms through immediate experience the power of spirituality in transforming our negative issues and enhancing our replacement positives. This is a vastly neglected part of the wholistic spectrum for many people.

As the age of science has progressed, explanations for aspects of nature have shown many religious teachings to be insupportable by scientific method. A prime example of this is the Biblical story of creation, which is contradicted by massive evidence from archeology, genetics, sociology, and anthropology. This has led many to abandon religion—and with it, spiritual awareness, as well as the belief that spiritual awareness is valid.

Now, however, people in modern Western society are redeveloping their spiritual lives through self-explorations with meditation, yoga, t'ai chi, qigong, communing with nature, and involvement in spiritual healing activities. There is also a return to religion as a pathway to spiritual awareness.

Many are coming to trust the inner gnowing that accompanies spiritual awareness. This is probably seen most dramatically in the transformations that occur with near-death and other strong mystical experiences. Less dramatic experiences, such as a moment of beauty or caring, can also be doorways into spiritual awakening. Spiritual healings commonly open into spiritual awareness. In fact, many healers suggest that illness, pains, and other forms of suffering may be stimuli from our higher selves to awaken us to our spirituality.

I make a distinction between spirituality and religion. Religion is for people who are afraid of going to hell; spirituality is for people who have been there.

—Timothy J. Mordaunt

WHEE invites people to open in many ways to their personal spiritual awareness:

- Raising the subject of spirituality for discussion in taking a history, prior to introducing WHEE, validates this "S-word" for people as a real and vital part of their life experiences.

- Using "and [God/Christ/the Infinite Source] loves and accepts me…" as part of counteracting positive affirmations and replacement affirmations invites people to have an immediate personal experience of the transformative power of spirituality in their lives. The incremental learning provided by WHEE is particularly helpful in this regard.

- Inviting the participation of the heart chakra and of Earth energies in the WHEE process provides immediate feedback on the potency of these energies in boosting self-healing through WHEE. By confirming these energetic components as part of the healing process, people become aware of themselves as energetic beings—not just physical beings.

- Helping people with WHEE through the proxy/surrogate method confirms that we are all interconnected—energetically and through the collective consciousness.

- Using muscle testing with a transpersonal focus invites people to explore their connections with other people and the greater world beyond their physical selves. Situations in which this is helpful may include: asking our unconscious mind to provide information about the states of other people (with their permission, of course); the suitability of a particular food item we want to eat; or any other information about the outer world that can give us feedback.

- Observing and acknowledging the magical synchronicities that occur in therapy and in other aspects of our lives is a way to raise awareness of our participation in the collective consciousness.

- Mirroring clients' experiences and beliefs, therapists can respectfully reflect back to clients the therapists' own spiritual presence. By being spiritually present, a therapist can help clients to resonate with the note of spirituality, thereby identifying and strengthening their own spiritual awareness. My own inclination is also to share carefully and selectively—from my beliefs, studies, and personal spiritual awareness—that which validates clients' beliefs and affirms their spiritual path as true (rather than imaginary).

- The process of offering intuitive awareness and proxy healing to clients is also a feedback to therapists regarding their own spiritual consciousness. The validations provided by clients can confirm the accuracy of therapists' intuitive perceptions and the effectiveness of their transpersonal interventions.

- Clients often provide lessons to therapists. The problems that they bring for treatment often resonate with similar problems the therapists can usefully address; their fortitude, dedication to personal growth and change, and overcoming of enormous loads of pain can be inspirational to therapists. My clients have often been some of my best teachers—in spirituality as in other levels of wholistic healing.

- The road to personal spiritual awareness often is marked by mental and emotional blocks and resistances. Many of these can be cleared by WHEE in the same manners that meta-issue resistances are addressed with other problems we want to clear. For instance, a common challenge in meditation is anxiety about letting go into the unstructured, unfamiliar territory of meditative awareness. Reducing this anxiety with WHEE can facilitate meditative focus.

- Past-life residues of unresolved emotional traumas can be cleared with WHEE. The experience of working through these issues can confirm experientially the validity of these memories. When the clearing of these past-life residues results in clearing of pain and other issues, there is reason to believe that these memories are as real as memories from current life traumas.

Several principles help to explain the effectiveness of WHEE beyond its benefits through mind-emotions-body healing. These are:

1. *Positives neutralize negatives.* Pairing the counteracting affirmation positive with a negative focus reduces the intensity of the negative. As long as it is a truly felt positive, it will be a potent tool for canceling any negativity. The same applies with installing replacement positives, which are then strengthened to be even more positive.

   The canceling of negatives with positives is a principle used in a variety of therapies.

   - Many of the *Energy Psychology* approaches use an affirmation positive similar to the ones suggested in this book.

   - *Behavior modification therapies* have developed several formats utilizing this principle.

   In *systematic desensitization,* people with fears and phobias are taught to enter a positive state such as relaxation, imagery, or meditation. They are then invited to relax prior to imagining themselves in an anxiety-provoking situation, starting at the mildest level of perceived stress. They ratchet up the tension in their imagination until it is moderately uncomfortable, at which point the then relax again. The positive mental state gradually cancels the anxiety.

In *flooding,* a similar method, people start at the maximal level of tension they can muster in their imagination around a problem, and then relax. Again, the positive cancels the negative.

- *Neurolinguistic Programming (NLP)* teaches the anchoring of a negative experience/fear/memory by pressing with a finger on one point on the body, anchoring a positive memory/feeling on another point on the body, and then pressing both points simultaneously. The positive diminishes the negative.

- *The presence of the therapist* is a universal positive that cancels negativity that is brought by a client to the session.

- *Installing the replacement positive* is another instance of this principle of positives that counteract negatives. Once a strong, positive opposite to the original negative focus is in place, it helps to neutralize further negatives of the same sort (that were eliminated by the WHEE process) when these are triggered by life events or by old habits.

2. *Staying with issues rather than running away from them* will initiate a clearing of the issues, in and of itself. When we overcome our childhood default of burying our problems and running away from them, we can deal with them in many ways.

- *The Sedona Method* has people focus on a negative issue, assess their SUDS, and ask themselves whether they are ready to release it. Just by holding the issue in awareness and giving ourselves permission to release it, the SUDS will go down. The same process works for installing the SUSS.

My personal impression is that the right-left alternating tapping and the affirmation both add significantly to this releasing process. I have also found that children (up to early teens) may not respond to the simple permission to release.

- *Rogerian therapy* has the therapist intervene primarily as a mirror to reflect back to the client what they are experiencing/saying/thinking/feeling. In addition to the presence of the therapist as an acknowledged healing factor, I am certain that holding issues in awareness without running away from them is also a healing factor.

- *Meditation* may be associated with "spontaneous" (i.e. unsought and unsolicited) releases of emotions. This phenomenon has no proven, nor any generally accepted hypothesized mechanisms to explain it. My personal opinion is that as people meditate and practice staying in the present moment, they also remain present and focused on negative issues as these arise. Staying focused on them and not running away will then spontaneously release the underlying, buried feelings.

3. *Sweetening spirals build more positives.* As we experience successes with WHEE, our self-confidence and self-image are enhanced. Because WHEE focuses on installing and strengthening positives (unlike many other therapies that focus mainly on addressing symptoms), it is a much more powerful and successful therapy.

   The replacement positive serves to help even more than just as a replacement for the negative focus. It is potent also because it stands on its own as a focus for building and strengthening sweetening spirals.

4. *Alternating right and left stimulation of the senses* (vision, hearing, touch, muscle tension/relaxation) stimulates and facilitates releases of physical and psychological pain, stress, anxiety, buried issues, and much more. This is a proven process, well documented clinically by EMDR and WHEE and validated in extensive research by EMDR, including impressive meta-analyses of series of EMDR studies. It is as yet a challenge to understand how this works. EMDR is seeking explanations through studies of neurophysiology, including the latest brain-imaging devices.

   My own simple explanation is a psychological one. As explained in Chapter 2, as children it is very helpful for us to run away from the hurt or to forget it; so, we bury the feelings outside of conscious awareness. In our earliest years, this is a good choice for dealing with pain and suffering, since we cannot avoid it. The problem is that we keep on hiding our feelings and running away from them out of habit—even though as adults we have many more and better options.

Our buried feeling memories are stored in unconscious portions of the right side of the brain. The right brain puts a sign on the locked closet, saying *"Keep away!"* It then turns to the left brain, where our conscious mind resides, and says, "We don't want to know about this, do we?" And the left brain says, "No, let's stay away from those painful memories and feelings." So we pretend to ourselves they aren't there.

When we stop running away from these buried feelings, holding them in our conscious mind and at the same time stimulating the right and left side of our body, we are activating the right and left sides of our brain. Holding our focus in this way is particularly powerful in releasing buried materials because we bring together the feelings and the awareness of the feelings that were split when the feelings were buried, and that continued to be held separated by the right and left brain hemispheres.

5. As mentioned before, WHEE is simple, easily learned, rapidly effective, user-friendly, and highly adaptive to individual preferences and needs.

Broader Understandings from WHEE

Learn why the world wags and what wags it. That is the only thing which the mind can never exhaust, never alienate, never be tortured by, never fear or distrust, and never dream of regretting.... Look what a lot of things there are to learn.

—Terence Hanbury White

Working on our pains and other life challenges with wholistic approaches, we deepen our awareness of every level of our being.

Our Body is Far More Than the Sum Total of Our Existence

Western medicine has made the body its primary focus, to the exclusion of most other levels of our being. WHEE demonstrates experientially that the body is intimately interconnected with the other levels of our wholistic spectrum of being. Most people can easily see that their mind and emotions are intimately linked with their body. What is experienced at one level is usually reflected at the other levels.

Our Life Is an Expression of Spirit and Soul

Intuition and spiritual awareness speak to us through our body. The feedback we get that validates intuitive awareness through muscle testing reinforces our trust in what our body tells us and in the reality of our intuitions—as they are validated through our life experiences.

When we extend our intuitive awareness to transpersonal issues, such as asking whether we will enjoy a blind date, we then get feedback on our participation in human collective consciousness. Asking through muscle testing whether an employment option or educational or career choice will turn out well, and observing the unfolding of our choice confirms our connection with the vaster collective consciousness of the cosmos.

As we begin to see that past-life experiences may be more than fantasies, we gain confidence that spirit and soul survive physical death. This may be one of the most deeply helpful aspects of spiritual awareness. When we do not fear death, life becomes a very different experience.

Eastern spiritual traditions teach that life is a much deeper experience than most people appreciate. Our individual lives are not just random genetic occurrences. Our soul chooses the family members, circumstances, and other relationships that will benefit its progress through the series of lifetime "classrooms" in which it is participating; and its spirit enters the body of a baby in utero to start the lessons of this particular life. Each lifetime provides precisely the right challenges that our soul needs for its growth and development.

From this perspective, all the challenges in our health, relationships, and careers are not just lessons to our physical selves that end with our physical death. We bring with us at birth the wisdom of experience and also the burdens of unresolved issues from previous lifetimes. We carry away with us after physical death the further accumulated lessons from our most recent lifetime.

Broadening the frame of reference through consultations with very gifted intuitives who can channel information from transpersonal dimensions, we find that people in family and friendship relationships in our current life often were related to us in previous lifetimes. This has been called karma—the balance sheet of positive and negative interactions we have brought with us from interactions with others over many lessons in uncounted classrooms. It is not uncommon to find when we have had experienced someone being difficult toward us in this lifetime that we have been difficult toward them in a previous lifetime. The challenges for each of us are to learn compassion and forgiveness.

Widening the lens further, karma is generated by families, cultural groups, nations, and by humanity as a whole. For instance, descendants of immigrant Americans and Canadians carry a karmic load from their ancestors' mistreatments of Native Americans.

WHEE can help us to release residues of feelings related to specific karmic relationships, as we become aware of them. We can use WHEE on these, in the same ways we would use WHEE on issues from our current lifetime.

We can also use generic clearing for such issues. We might include the following in a setup focus: *"I hereby release all..."*

- "...residues of anxieties, fears, and pains on any and all levels of my awareness from injuries I sustained in my [identify body parts] in any and all previous lifetimes..."

- "...hurts, angers, resentments, and wishes for revenge from any and all previous lifetimes in my relationship with [name/relationship], and I love and accept myself..."

- "...jealousies and possessiveness from any and all previous lifetimes in my relationship with [name/relationship]..."

WHEE clients have sometimes experienced surprising shifts in physical and emotional pains and other symptoms from using such generic affirmations with spiritual focus.[1]

My personal belief is that my life is a role chosen by my soul for my personal lessons and advancement and for the lessons and advancement of others with whom I interact. As a pixel on the big screen I do my best to clear the dross of hurts, fears, and angers within me and around me so that the screen can be brighter and clearer. WHEE has been an enormous help to me and to others in these ways. I hope WHEE will be helpful to you in these ways, as well.

---

[1] For further discussions on the interrelationships between body, emotions, mind, relationships and spirits, click on the round icons at www.wholistichealingresearch. com. Questions about even deeper meanings of life are beyond the scope of this book. See discussions in *Healing Research, Volume III: Personal Spirituality.*

Extending WHEE into the Collective Consciousness

Humanity is destroying our planet and is thereby suiciding. These are behaviors of a collective PTSD. Just as individuals who suffered abuse tend to become violent, to abuse others and to suicide, humanity as a collective is doing the same. This PTSD is turning people into perpetrators of further violence and of planetary destruction. If humanity can clear the angers, fears and hurts perpetuating our PTSD, we may be able to cooperate with each other in solving problems of carbon emissions, global heating, pollution and wasted resources – all of which may soon reach tipping points beyond which there is no return from a path to planetary destruction.

Here are approaches that might help this collective PTSD:

1. WHEE can help us clear ourselves so that each of us becomes a brighter and clearer pixel on the big world screen. We can encourage others to do the same.

2. To address the collective homicidal and suicidal madness of mankind, we can add invitations for healing post-traumatic stress throughout the collective consciousness of our planet as we engage in any therapy and healing processes (personally or as therapists). For instance, after using WHEE on myself or with others, I offer this silent invitation for collective consciousness healing: "I invite anyone and everyone, anywhere and everywhere, anywhen and everywhen to clear whatever issues they have that resonate with my/our clearing." I invite others to do whatever might feel right to you along these lines.

Maybe, just maybe, we can heal the collective PTSD of humanity that perpetuates the cycles of being abused → hurt → anger → perpetrating abuse on others → etc.

Healing through the collective consciousness is limited only by our beliefs and disbeliefs. We could extend this healing intent to all generations back to our common genetic ancestor, the mythical 'Lucy,' and beyond. We might even invite clearing for whatever and whomever might have brought her to be the survivor of some tragedy that wiped out all other genetic lines.

I'd be pleased to have your feedback on how these approaches work for you, and to hear any healing suggestions you might have.

Afterword:
Looking to a New Future

The future enters us long before we're aware of it.

— Rilke

Our world is in crisis. Humans have not found the ways to live harmoniously in large groups. Accumulation of wealth and power are the goals that Western society, the dominant social model on our planet, has promoted — individually and collectively. We pursue local self-interests, and greedy, powerful nations and multinational corporations amass resources for themselves at the expense of less powerful nations and groups. This is producing scarcities of vital resources and conflicts between nations and between subcultures within nations. Political leaders are lighting and fanning flames of fears to manipulate and divert people from dealing with the critical issues of dwindling resources and the pollution by industries that are producing global heating. ("Warming" is an unacceptable euphemism!)

When will our consciences grow so tender that we will act to prevent human misery rather than avenge it?

— Eleanor Roosevelt

Reducing levels of stress more widely could provide ways to remove the kindling that is so easily set ablaze. Venting angers collectively on "others" does nothing more than create and perpetuate excuses for wars. If we pursue a policy of "an eye for an eye," then pretty soon everyone will be blind.

Imagine a future where…

- WHEE and other self-healing methods are taught from pre-school up;

- Children grow up without running away from their pains and fears;

- Angers are dissipated quickly and easily, allowing any underlying hurts and fears to surface and be cleared, too;

- Traumas, even severe ones, are experienced as invitations to learn more about ourselves, and post-traumatic stress disorders are a thing of the past;

- Building sweetening spirals is a daily exercise;

- Vicious circles never have a chance to take root;

- Perpetrators of sexual and physical abuse are offered WHEE to clear residues of their own childhood abuses that are being expressed through re-enacting their traumas upon others;

- Correctional facilities teach WHEE so that inmates can release the hurts, angers, depression, and addictions that contributed to their incarceration;

- People in high-stress jobs use WHEE to de-stress, thereby improving the atmosphere in the workplace, decreasing stress-related illness and absenteeism;

- WHEE is used as a treatment of first choice for pain and stress-related illnesses, thereby reducing the need for medications and saving lives;

- Wholistic healing is the prevalent approach to health care, offering the best of all worlds to everyone;

- Collective levels of fears and angers are lessened, thereby decreasing conflicts between individuals, families, communities, and nations…

> *World peace must develop from inner peace.*
> *Peace is not the absence of violence.*
> *Peace is the manifestation of compassion.*
>
> —His Holiness The Dalai Lama

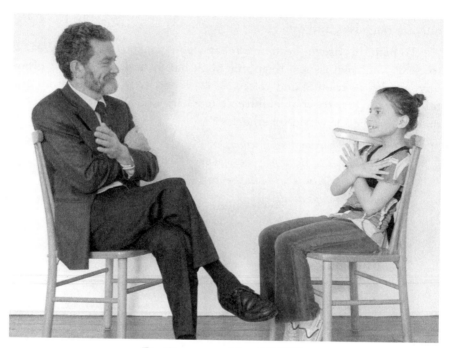

Dr. Benor teaching WHEE.

I envision a world in which children know from personal experience that the world is a good place to live and that anything at all that happens to them will be okay in the end. In other words, a world that is without fears.

Without fears, we are not as easily swayed by demagogues in politics, religion, or the corporate sphere who, driven by motivations of power and greed, would have us bend our backs to serve their wishes. Nor do we invest our energies or resources in wars, choosing instead to nurture ourselves and others.

To help this dream become a reality, you can start by using WHEE to clear your own issues. Keep this book handy and use WHEE often. Give copies to friends and relatives; send copies to your doctors and other caregivers, to your children's teachers and your mentors. Let's make this a better world together!

> *Hope is the thing with feathers*
> *that perches in the soul*
> *and sings the tune without the words*
> *and never stops at all.*

> —Emily Dickinson

Suggested Reading

Bair, Christine Caldwell. *The heart field effect: synchronization of healer-subject heart rates in energy therapy*, (Dissertation) Holos University Graduate Seminary, Springfield, MO, in partial fulfillment of the requirements for the degree of Doctor of Theology 2006.

Bair, Christine Caldwell. Research confirming WHEE is helpful. Summary at: www.wholistichealingresearch.com/WHEE_Research. html; Download copy of dissertation at http://holosuniversity.net/ abstracts.asp#bair

Benor, Daniel J. WHEE introductory article. www.wholistic healingresearch.com/Articles/Selfheal.asp

Benor, Daniel J. WHEE for trauma and re-entry problems. www. heal911.com/C-6a.asp

Benor, Daniel J. WHEE for children of all ages. www.wholistic healingresearch.com/Articles/WHEE-Child.asp

Benor, Daniel J. The inter-relationships of spirit, relationships (with people and the environment, mind, emotions and body. www.wholistic healingresearch.com/srmeb.htm

Benor, Daniel J. (See list of books, below.)

Berne, Eric. *Games People Play*. New York, NY: Random House 1996

Capacchione, Lucia. *Recovery of Your Inner Child: The Highly Acclaimed Method for Liberating Your Inner Self*. New York, NY: Fireside 1991.

Caudill, Margaret. *Managing Pain Before It Manages You*. New York, NY: Guilford 2002.

Chaitow, Leon. *Conquer Pain the Natural Way: A Practical Guide*. San Francisco, CA: Chronicle Books 2002.

Clinton, Asha Nahoma. *The Seemorg Core Belief Matrices & Protocol: almost all the cognitions you'll evern need to work with*. http://seemorg matrix.org/HomePages/Market.html

Cohen, Darlene. *Turning Suffering Inside Out: A Zen Approach to Living with Physical and Emotional Pain*. Boston, MA: Shambhala 2000.

Cohen, Kenneth S. *Honoring the Medicine: Native American Healing*. New York, NY: Ballantine 2003.

Davies, Clair, Davies, Amber, and Simons, David. *The Trigger Point Therapy Workbook: Your Self-Treatment Guide for Pain Relief*. 2nd Ed. Oakland, CA: New Harbinger 2004.

Davis, Laura. *Allies in Healing*. New York, NY: HarperPerennial 1991. (The first is for people with history of sexual, physical, emotional abuse, the second for partners of same. Outstanding discussion, with heavy but helpful case materials. For therapists and laypersons.)

Davis, Laura and Bass, Ellen. *Beginning to Heal: A First Book for Survivors of Child Sexual Abuse*. New York, NY: HarperPerennial 1993.

Dienstfrey, Harris. *Where the Mind Meets the Body*. New York, NY: HarperPerennial 1991. (Good discussion of Psychoneuroimmunology.)

Dennison, P. E./Dennison, G. E. *Brain Gym: Teachers Edition, Revised*. Ventura, CA: Edu-Kinesthetics 1994.

Dennison, P. E., and Dennison, G. E. *Brain Gym Handbook*. Ventura, CA: Educational Kinesiology Foundation 1989.

Dethlefson, Thorwald, and Dahlke, Rudiger. *The Healing Power of Illness: The Meaning of Symptoms and How to Interpret Them*. Longmead, UK: Element 1990 (Orig. German 1983).

Dillard, James. *The Chronic Pain Solution: Your Personal Path to Pain Relief*. New York, NY: Bantam 2002.

Egoscue, Pete. *Pain Free: A Revolutionary Method for Stopping Chronic Pain*. New York, NY: Bantam 1998.

Eimer, Bruce. *Hypnotic Yourself Out of Pain Now*. Oakland, CA: New Harbinger 2002.

Epstein, Gerald. *Healing Visualizations: Creating Health Through Imagery.* New York/London: Bantam 1989.

Feinstein, David. Energy psychology in disaster relief. www. EnergyTraumaTreatment.com

David Feinstein, PhD. *Energy Psychology Interactive: Rapid Interventions for Lasting Change.* Ashland, OR: Innersource 2004.

Feinstein, David, Eden, Donna and Craig, Gary. *The Promise of Energy Psychology: Revolutionary Tools for Dramatic Personal Change.* New York, NY: Tarcher/Penguin 2005.

Goleman, Daniel/Gurin, Joel. *Mind Body Medicine.* Yonkers, New York, NY: Consumer Reports 1993. (Well-referenced review.)

Hawken. Paul. *Blessed Unrest: How the Largest Movement in the World Came into Being and Why No One Saw it Coming,* NY: Viking/Penguin 2007.

Hay, Louise L. *You Can Heal Your Life.* Santa Monica, CA: Hay House 1984.

Hirschberg, Caryl, and Barasch, Marc Ian. *Remarkable Recovery: What Extraordinary Healings Tell Us About Getting Well and Staying Well.* New York: Riverhead 1995. (Excellent descriptions of personal transformations through illness.)

Laing, Ronald D. *Knots.* New York, NY: Penguin 1970.

Goleman, Daniel, and Gurin, Joel (eds.). *Mind-Body Medicine: How to Use Your Mind for Better Health.* New York, NY: Consumer Reports 1993.

Harrison, John. *Love Your Disease — It's Keeping You Healthy.* London, UK: Angus and Robertson 1984.

Ingram, Catherine. *Passionate Presence: Experiencing the Seven Qualities of Awakened Awareness.* New York, NY: Gotham Books, 2003.

LeShan, Lawrence. *You Can Fight for Your Life: Emotional Factors in the Treatment of Cancer.* New York, NY: M. Evans 1977.

LeShan, Lawrence. *Cancer as a Turning Point.* New York, NY: E. P. Dutton 1989.

Levine, Peter. *Healing Trauma: A Pioneering Program for Restoring the Wisdom of Your Body.* Boulder, CO: Sounds True (audio) 2005.

Levine, Peter. *Waking the Tiger: Healing Trauma*. Berkeley, CA: North Atlantic Books 1997.

Levine, Peter, and Kline, Maggie. *Trauma Through A Child's Eyes*. Berkeley, CA: North Atlantic Books 2007.

Levine, Stephen. *Who Dies? An Investigation of Conscious Living and Conscious Dying*. Bath, England: Gateway 1986.

Levine, Stephen. *Unattended Sorrow: Recovering from Loss and Reviving the Heart*. New York, NY: Rodale 2005.

May, Gerald. *Grace and Addiction: Lore and Spirituality in the Healing of Addictions*. San Francisco, CA: Harper 2007.

May, Gerald. *The Wisdom of Wilderness: Experiencing the Healing Powers of Nature*. San Francisco: Harper 2006.

Melzack, Ronald, and Wall, Patrick. *The Challenge of Pain*. 2nd Edition. New York, NY: Bantam 2004.

Naparstek, Belleruth. *Invisible Heroes: Survivors of Trauma and How They Heal*. New York, NY: Bantam 2004.

Ogden, Pat, Minton, Kekuni, and Pain, Clare. *Trauma and the Body: A Sensorimotor Approach to Psychotherapy*. New York, NY: Norton 2006.

O'Regan, Brendan/ Hirshberg, Caryle. *Spontaneous Remission: An Annotated Bibliography*. Sausalito, CA: Institute of Noetic Sciences 1993.

Paul, Margaret. *Inner Bonding: Becoming a Loving Adult to Your Inner Child*. San Francisco, CA: HarperSanFrancisco 1992.

Phillips, Maggie, Dennison, P. E. and Dennison, G. E. *Brain Gym Handbook*. Ventura, CA: Educational Kinesiology Foundation 1989/2000.

Phillips, Maggie. Hypnosis with depression, posttraumatic stress disorder, and chronic pain. pp. 217–241 in Michael Yapko (ed.), *Hypnosis and Treating Depression: Applications in Clinical Practice*. New York, NY: Routledge 2006.

Rossi, Ernest. *The Psychobiology of Mindbody Healing: New Concepts of Therapeutic Hypnosis*. New York, NY: Norton 1997.

Roud, Paul C. *Making Miracles: An Exploration into the Dynamics of Self-Healing*. Wellingborough, England: Thorsons 1990. (People who were successful at self-healing tell their stories.)

Sheikh, A. A. (ed). *Imagination and Healing.* Farmingdale, New York, NY: Baywood 1984. (Visualizations—theoretical discussion.)

Siegel, Bernie S. *Love, Medicine & Miracles: Lessons Learned About Self-Healing from a Surgeon's Experience with Exceptional Patients.* New York, NY: Harper & Row 1986.

Siegel, Bernie. Respants: Information, Inspiration and Expiration. *International J. of Healing and Caring—On line.* www.ijhc.org 2002, 2(1), 1–5.

Simonton, O. C. et al. *Getting Well Again.* Los Angeles, CA: Tarcher 1978. (Self-healing for cancer.)

Spear, Deena Zalkind. *Ears of the Angels.* Carlsbad, CA: Hay House, Inc., 2002.

Spiegel, David et al. Effect of Psychosocial Treatment on Survival of Patients with Metastatic Breast Cancer. *Lancet.* No. 8668, ii (1989). (Cancer support groups.)

Steadman, A. *Who's the Matter with Me?* Marina del Rey, CA: DeVorss 1966.

Stewart, Ian and Joines, Vann. *TA Today.* Chapel Hill, NC: Lifespace 1991.

Tolle, Eckhart, *The Power of Now: A Guide to Spiritual Enlightenment.* Novato, CA: New World 1999.

Tolle, Eckhart. *A New Earth: Awakening to Your Life's Purpose.* New York, NY: Plume/Penguin 2006.

Tolle, Eckhart. Dissolving the pain body. http://commonground.ca/iss/051017/cg171_tolle.shtml

Transactional Analysis Websites: www.businessballs.com/transactional analysis.htm; http://en.wikipedia.or/wiki/Transactional_analysis

Turk, Dennis, and Nash, Justin. Chronic pain: New ways to cope. pp. 111-130 in Daniel Goleman & Joel Gurin (eds), *Mind-Body Medicine.* New York, NY: Consumer Reports Books 1993.

Turk, Dennis, and Winter, Frits. *The Pain Survival Guide: How to Reclaim Your Life.* Washington, DC: American Psychological Association 2006.

Whitfield, C.L. *Healing the Child Within: Discovery and Recovery for Adult Children of Dysfunctional Families.* Health Communications 1989.

Wright, Machaelle Small. *Co-Creative Science: A Revolution In Science Providing Real Solutions For Today's Health & Environment.* Warrenton, VA: Perelandra, Ltd. 1997.

Zeig, Jeffrey, and Geary, B. Ericksonian approaches to pain management. pp. 252–262 in Geary & Zeig (eds.). *The Handbook of Ericksonian Psychotherapy.* Phoenix, AZ: The Milton H. Erickson Foundation 2001.

See also list of books, tapes and other Meridian Based Therapy references: www.wholistichealingreasearch.com/References/MBTs.htm

EMDR

Shapiro, Francine. *Eye Movement Desensitization and Reprocessing.* New York, NY: Guildford 1995.
www.emdr.com

EMDR for Children

Greenwald, Ricky. Eye movement desensitization and reprocessing (EMDR): New hope for children suffering from trauma and loss. www.childtrauma.com/emdrch.html

Research References
EMDR
www.emdr.com/efficacy.htm

EFT

Feinstein, David. Energy psychology: A review of the preliminary evidence. *Psychotherapy: Theory, Research, Practice, Training.* (in press) www.innersource.net/energy_psych/epi_research.htm

Parapsychology and Reincarnation

Kelsey, Denys/Grant, Joan. *Many Lifetimes.* Garden City, NY: Doubleday 1967.

Lawrence, Tony. Bringing home the sheep: a meta-analysis of sheep/goat experiments. *Proceedings of 36ᵗʰ Annual Parapsychology Convention 1993*. Fairhaven, MA: Parapsychological Association.

Radin, Dean. *The Conscious Universe*. New York: HarperCollins 1997.

Radin D. I. and Ferrari D. C. Effects of consciousness on the fall of dice: A meta-analysis. *Journal of Scientific Exploration*. 1991, 5, 61–84.

Radin D./Nelson, R. Meta-analysis of mind-matter interaction experiments: 1959 to 2000; www.boundaryinstitute.org/articles/rngma.pdf (Accessed 2/26/06.)

Stevenson, Ian. *Children Who Remember Previous Lives: A Question of Reincarnation*. Charlottesville, VA: University of Virginia 1987.

Wambach, Helen. *Life Before Life*. New York: Bantam 1979.

Energy Psychology Modalities (a few of many)

Allergy Antidotes — Sandra Kost Radomski, ND, LCSW
www.allergy antidotes.com

Emotional Freedom Technique (EFT) — Gary Craig
www.emofree.com

Healing from the Body Level Up (HBLU) — Judith A. Swack, PhD
www.jaswack.com/

Seemorg Matrix Therapy — Asha Nahoma Clinton
http://seemorgmatrix.org

Tapas Acupressure Technique (TAT) — Tapas Fleming
www.tatlife.com

Related references by Daniel J. Benor

Healing Research: Volume 1, Spiritual Healing: Scientific Validation of a Healing Revolution. Southfield, MI: Vision Publications, 2001. (Healers describe their work, research in parapsychology as a context for understanding healing, brief summaries of randomized controlled studies, pilot studies.)

Healing Research: Volume 1, Professional Supplement. Southfield, MI: Vision Publications, 2001. (Only the studies — described in much greater detail, including statistical information.)

Healing Research, Volume 2 (Popular edition): How Can I Heal What Hurts? Medford, NJ: Wholistic Healing Publications, 2005. (Written for the layperson. Same content as Professional edition but minus the masses of research references; plus extra chapter on Self-Healing approaches.)

Healing Research, Volume 2 (Professional edition): Consciousness, Bioenergy and Healing. Medford, NJ: Wholistic Healing Publications, 2004. (Self-healing, wholistic complementary/alternative medicine and integrative care, biological energies, and environmental interactions with bioenergies. *Consciousness, Bioenergy, and Healing* was acknowledged as "Book of the Year" by the Scientific and Medical Network, UK.)

Healing Research, Volume 3: Personal Spirituality: Science, Spirit and the Eternal Soul. Medford, NJ: Wholistic Healing Publications 2006. (Research on NDE, OBE, spirit survival, reincarnation, spiritual awareness.)

Reaching Higher and Deeper: Workbook for Healing Research, Volume 3: Personal Spirituality. Bellmawr, NJ: Wholistic Healing Publications 2007.

Healing Research, Volume 4—A Synthesis of Recent Research. Medford, NJ: Wholistic Healing Publications (in press). (Topical summaries of Volumes 1–3, with discussion of theories, early synthesis of explanations for healing; in press.)

Spiritual healing for mental health. In: Shannon, Scott (ed). *Handbook of Complementary and Alternative Therapies in Mental Health.* San Diego, CA: Academic/Harcourt 2001, 258–267. www.WholisticHealingResearch.com/Articles/MentalHlth-SpirHeal.htm

Spiritual healing for infertility, pregnancy, labor and delivery. *Complementary Therapies in Nursing and Midwifery.* 1996, 2, 106–109.

Psychotherapy & spiritual healing. *Human Potential.* 1996 (summer), 13–16.

Further comments on "loading" and "telesomatic reactions." *Advances.* 1996, 12(2), 71–75.

Spiritual Healing: A unifying influence in complementary therapies. *Complementary Therapies in Medicine.* 1995, 3(4), 234–238.

Spiritual healing and psychotherapy. *The Therapist.* 1994, 1(4), 37–39, www.wholistichealingresearch.com/spiritualhealingandpsychotherapy.html

Intuitive assessments: An overview. www.wholistichealingresearch
.com/intuitiveassessmentsoverview.html

Intuitive diagnosis. *Subtle Energies*. 1992, 3(2), 41–64, www.wholistic
healingresearch.com/IntuitiveAssessPilot.html

A psychiatrist examines fears of healing. *J. Society for Psychical Research*.
1990, 56, 287–299, www.wholistichealingresearch.com/psychiatrist
examines.html

Fields and energies related to healing: A review of Soviet & western
studies. *Psi Research*. 1984, 3(1), 8–15. Reprinted in *International
Journal of Healing and Caring*, January, 2004, 4(1), 1–12.

The overlap of psychic "readings" with psychotherapy. *Psi Research*.
1986, 5(1,2), 56–78.

**See many more articles by Dr. Benor at www.wholistichealing
research.com/articles.html**

Glossary

Acupressure — Pressure applied at acupuncture points for relief of symptoms and illnesses.

Affirmation — Positive statement that is made as one focuses on a negative feeling or thought. The positive counteracts and neutralizes the negative. (Not to be confused with the *replacement positive statement*, defined below.)

Clairsentience — Knowledge about an animate or inanimate object, without the use of sensory cues (sometimes called psychometry or remote viewing). This may appear in the mind of the perceiver as visual imagery (clairvoyance), auditory messages (clairaudience), or other *internal* sensory awareness, such as taste, smell, or a mirroring of bodily sensations from another person.

Concern — an appropriate need expressed without emotional attachments.

Core beliefs — Beliefs that we usually installed in our unconscious minds when we were young, at a time when we uncritically accepted them because we were just at the stage of absorbing what the world is about. Examples: "I could never be loved." "I am [clumsy/dumb/ugly/unable to be understood/and so on]."

Emotional Freedom Technique (EFT) — A therapy in which you tap or press a finger at a series of acupressure points on your face, chest, and hand, while reciting an affirmation.

Energy Psychology — A group of methods that include tapping or pressing on acupressure points and chakras as part of the therapy, with or without affirmations. Modalities include TFT, EFT, TAT, Seemorg Matrix Therapy, and many others. Often used synonymously with Meridian Based Therapies.

ESP—See *Extrasensory Perception.*

Extrasensory Perception—Telepathy, clairsentience, pre- and retro-cognition.

Eye Movement Desensitization and Reprocessing (EMDR)—A very simple but very potent technique that involves alternating right and left stimulation of the body, back and forth, while focusing on feelings (often attached to an experience or issue) that one would like to change. Doing EMDR repeatedly can reduce and eliminate negative feelings and install positive ones.

Faith—Belief without preliminary factual basis in the material world; also a meta-belief in the validity of another belief.

Focusing statement—See *Setup statement.*

Gaia—The ecobiological system consisting of the planet Earth and everything on it, living and non-living, that exists in a homeostatic state of balance in which conditions for life as we know it are maintained over the millennia.

Gnosis/Gnowing—Direct, intuitive knowledge that often carries with it an inner, numinous sense of certainty about its validity. This is an awareness through the intuitive right brain for some; for others it is a knowing felt in the heart rather than in the head. To those who have experienced gnosis, it may feel even more real than physical reality, which, in comparison, is sometimes described as an illusion.

Healing—See *spiritual healing.* (Used in this context as distinct from the physical processes of healing from injury or illness.)

Intuition—Thought without underlying logical basis. The use of intuition alone does not imply that facts were gathered with other than the five usual senses. Intuition, of itself, is neutral and not necessarily spiritual. One can think intuitively about science or mathematics, for example. Intuition can have several layers, including:

- pattern recognition based on pervious experiences with situations that are similar to the current one

- psychic (extrasensory/psi) impressions deriving from telepathy, clairsentience, pre- and retrocognition

- bioenergy perceptions acquired through interactions of one person's biological energy field(s) with the field(s) of other living beings and non-living things

- spiritual awareness, derived from transpersonal consciousness

Karma—The unresolved feelings and relationships that we return to work through in future lifetimes when we do not complete the clearing in the lifetime when the negativity was generated.

Meridians—Biological energy lines identified many thousands of years ago by acupuncture. Along these lines are sensitive points that can be stimulated to facilitate flows or release blocks of bioenergies in the body, thereby clearing symptoms and illnesses and promoting health.

Meridian Based Therapy (MBT)—See *Energy Psychology.*

Meta-anxieties—Anxieties about other, primary issues. Meta-anxieties block us from dealing with the primary issues. Example: "If I let myself feel *x* fully, I will be overwhelmed." See also *Core beliefs.*

Muscle testing—Inviting the unconscious mind to respond to questions through muscle responses.

Psi (Psychic or Extra Sensory Perception)—Thought or experience based on information or sensory inputs gathered without the use of the five usual senses, including telepathy, clairsentience, precognition, and retrocognition. Once within the unconscious or conscious mind, this information may be processed in a logical way, or may be handled intuitively. Psi perceptions are not inherently good or bad any more than perceptions based on our physical senses are. Psi may represent the most primitive or generalized form of knowing. Indications are that it is often an inherited capacity and can improve with use. It can also be a learned skill, as most people have some measure of psi ability. Examples: auric vision, telepathy, remote viewing, psychometry, psychokinesis (PK).

Replacement positive statement—WHEE (like EMDR) invites you to install a positive statement to replace a negative feeling or thought that you have released, after the SUDS is down to zero.

Round—A round of WHEE involves tapping on an issue after checking the SUDS or SUSS, then checking the SUDS or SUSS again to see how much the negative has been released, or how much the counteracting positive has been strengthened.

Secondary gain—Rewards associated with the expression of pain may influence the frequency of its occurrence and the severity of its expression.

Series—As many rounds of WHEE as are needed from the initial negative point to the final positive point.

Setup (focusing) statement—The precise statement used in starting a round of WHEE, including all the psychological and physical feelings with the associated thoughts and memories.

Shadow—Those parts of our unconscious mind that we would rather not be aware of, including major and minor traumatic experiences, feelings which we find uncomfortable, self-doubts and misgivings we would rather not perceive, and the like.

Soul—That part of a person that survives death and integrates aspects of the person's most recent personality with their eternal Self. (Some prefer to call this part the *spirit*. See also *spirit* for my explanation of my preference for *soul* here and *spirit* there.)

Spirit—That part of a person that survives death and still retains aspects of the person's personality. (Some prefer to call this part the *soul*. I prefer *spirit* because of the popular use of this term to denote those who have passed on but return to communicate through channeled messages or as apparitions. See also *Soul*.)

Spiritual gifts (sitvas, charisms)—Extraordinary abilities that may be acquired suddenly or as a result of spiritual practices, such as prolonged meditation or vision quests. For example: healing through touch or at a distance, prophesy, discernment of discarnate spirits, levitation, bilocation.

Spiritual healing—A systematic, purposeful intervention by one or more persons intending to help another living being (person, animal, plant, or other living system) by means of focused intention, hand contact, or movements of the hands around the body to improve their condition. Spiritual healing is brought about without the use of conventional energetic, mechanical, or chemical interventions. Some healers attribute spiritual healing occurrences to God, Christ, other "higher powers," spirits, universal or cosmic forces or energies, biological healing energies or forces residing in the healer, psychokinesis (mind over matter), or self-healing powers or energies latent in the healee. Psychological interventions are inevitably part of spiritual healing (as they are with every clinical intervention), but spiritual healing adds many dimensions to interpersonal healing factors.

Spirituality—Transpersonal awareness that arises spontaneously or through meditative and other practices, which are beyond ordinary explanations, and to which are attributed an inspiring and guiding meaningfulness, often attributed to a Deity. Spirituality has many facets. It is an individual's basic quest or understanding of ultimate meanings and values in life. Spirituality often results from primary experience, *gnosis*, which may be stimulated by strongly positive, traumatic, or transformational life occurrences, such as having to deal with pain; dramatic loss and grief; near death experiences, bereavement apparitions and channeled encounters with spirits; psychic or even psychotic episodes; and other encounters beyond ordinary experience. These may include healing crises and transformations. Spirituality often includes a sense of participating in a reality that is vaster than can be comprehended by human awareness, that is self-aware, totally loving and unconditionally accepting.

Subjective Units of Distress Scale (SUDS)—Rating scale from zero (not bothering you at all) to 10 (the worst it could possibly feel). Prior to and following each round of WHEE, it is helpful to assess how strong the negative feeling is that you are addressing.

SUDS—See *Subjective Units of Distress Scale.*

Subjective Units of Success Scale (SUSS)—Prior to beginning to install the replacement positive, and after each round of WHEE to strengthen it, you will find it helpful to check how strongly you believe and feel the replacement positive statement to be true, where zero is "not at all" and 10 is "it couldn't be stronger or firmer."

SUSS—See *Subjective Units of Success Scale.*

Sweetening spiral—When a positive action produces a positive response, which encourages further positive actions, and so on. The opposite of a *vicious circle.*

Synchronicity—Meaningful coincidences that appear to suggest a hidden or guiding order of collective awareness in the world.

Telepathy—The transfer of thoughts, images, or commands from one mind to another.

Traditional societies — Non-industrial societies in which there are unbroken traditions of personal spiritual awareness and healing.

Transactional analysis (TA) — Eric Berne's three basic *ego states*: Inner Parent, Adult and Child, which explain many of the ways people (regardless of our age) respond in various situations.

Transcendent — Relating to realities that are perceived as being outside of the physical world (but may include the physical), associated with a consciousness that is vastly higher and wiser than that of humanity.

Transpersonal — Awareness that extends beyond the body, often associated with feelings of being in touch with spiritual dimensions.

Worry — a concern with emotional overlays.

Names Index

Subject Index

"C" = case illustration or affirmation   "E" = exercise   "Def" = definition

About the Author

Daniel J. Benor, MD, ABIHM, has been searching over four decades for ever more ways to peel the onion of life's resistances, to reach the gnowing (with the inner knowing of truth which has the feel of rightness) that we are all cells in the body of the Infinite Source.

His principal work is through wholistic healing—addressing spirit, relationships, mind, emotions, and body. He teaches WHEE, a potent self-healing method, for adults and children who are dealing with psychological and physical pain, stress, PTSD, cravings, and other issues.

Dr. Benor founded The Doctor-Healer Networks in England and in North America. He authored of *Healing Research, Vol. 1–3* and many articles on wholistic healing. He is the editor of the International Journal of Healing and Caring (www.ijhc.org) and moderator of a major informational website on spiritual awareness, healing, and CAM research (www.WholisticHealingResearch.com).

Dr. Benor appears internationally on radio and TV. He is a Founding Diplomat of the American Board of Integrative Holistic Medicine; Founder and Past Coordinator for the Council for Healing (www.councilforhealing.org); and has served for many years on the advisory boards of the journals *Alternative Therapies, Subtle Energies, Frontier Sciences, Explore;* the Advisory Council of the Association for Comprehensive Energy Psychotherapy (ACEP), Emotional Freedom Techniques (EFT), and the Advisory Board of the Research Council for Complementary Medicine (UK). Dr. Benor teaches WHEE in lectures, workshops and teleseminars.

See www.WholisticHealingResearch.com; www.ijhc.org; www.paintap.com; E-mail: DB@WholisticHealingResearch.com